The BodySpeak™ Manual

Moving Body and Mind

A collection of writings and exercises for developing kinesthetic intelligence

Exploring the philosophy and practice
of Body*Speak* ™ training

by

Samuel Avital

with an INTRODUCTION and AFTERWORD by Jane Evenson

and a FOREWORD by Mark Olsen

ISBN: 0-75962-699-5

This book is printed on acid free paper.

This publication is directed to those who genuinely inquire
and for those interested in Body*Speak*™ training, classes,
seminars, and private consultations.

Le Centre du Silence Mime School
Information Center
P.O. Box 1015
Boulder, Colorado 80306
savital@concentric.net

1stBooks – rev. 04/26/01

"Though Aristotle spoke of dancers who need neither poetry nor music, and such famous choreographers as Noverre, Folkine, Diaghilev, and Balanchine have used mimetic invention in ballet, the illusive art of mime did not come to America until Marceau brought it in 1955. It has grown in importance ever since.

"...Samuel Avital, Director of Le Centre Du Silence Mime School, is one of the most interesting persons now teaching mime (and more). His *Mime Work Book* and *Mime & Beyond: The Silent Outcry,* originally written and used by Avital in the classroom, is now being read by teachers, actors, clowns, mimes, and dancers from coast to coast. **Universal in appeal,** it glows with Avital's personality."

American Dance Guild Book Club

"'A fool cannot feel,' said the Hebrew sages. If a man does not feel he cannot sense differences, and of course he will not be able to distinguish between one action and another. Without this ability to differentiate there can be no learning, and certainly no increase in the ability to learn. It is not a simple matter, for the human senses are linked to the stimuli that produce them so that discrimination is finest when the stimulus is smallest.

"If I raise an iron bar I shall not feel the difference if a fly either lights on it or leaves it. If, on the other hand, I am holding a feather, I shall feel a distinct difference if the fly were to settle on it. The same applies to all the senses: hearing, sight, smell, taste, heat, and cold."

Moshe Feldenkrais, *Awareness Through Movement*

DEDICATION

This book is dedicated in homage and with profound honor
to all my beloved teachers, women and men on all planes of existence,
who took what was offered,
and who gave what could not be taken.

Samuel Avital, January 2nd, 2001

ACKNOWLEDGMENTS

I would like to give thanks to the beautiful people I have encountered during my teaching. And, to those close to me who were dedicated to learning and sharing from their source of knowledge to teach me a thing or two, for which I am very grateful.

In particular to the untiring efforts and attention to detail, directed focus and care of Jane Evenson, my good friend and the "Englishizer" of my words. I call Jane the "word acrobat." She sculpts, forms, and shapes the words. Jane's introduction and the afterword for this book are works of art that explore the kinesthetic intelligence in the Body*Speak*™ method, revealing the active dimension of this work. I appreciate knowing you and being with you. With my full gratitude, thank you for being here.

To Alessandra, my dedicated student and friend, who loves to learn and apply the teachings. She typed, edited and arranged the Creative Body*Speak*™ Exercises section in this book, which she actively practiced over the years. I am grateful to you for your unceasing devotion, focused attention and caring assistance. With my full gratitude, thank you for being here.

To Mark Olsen, my student and friend who applied and practiced and made my teachings his own, adapting them to his life needs. Among other articles he has written about my work, he has composed the eloquent and beautiful foreword to this Body*Speak*™ *Manual*. Thank you for being here.

To Penny Collins for her input on the graphics for the text and to C. D. Miles-Yepez for his dedicated work in finalizing and formatting the book. My sincere appreciation.

To all my beloved students over the years who taught me humility, persistence, and the love of teaching and gently transmitting. Wherever you are, I give you my profound thanks and send you my warmest love.

And, finally to my beloved family—my grandfather, my father, my mother, my aunt Rachel, the Cosmic Jester of my hometown in Sefrou, Morocco, my brothers and sisters and their beautiful families— and to my cherished extended family in the United States, the Evensonian Galaxy. All and more have formed me and sustained me. To all of you, visibly and invisibly, I thank you humbly for your loving presence.

TABLE OF CONTENTS

FOREWARD

By Mark Olsen

There's an old saying that if you want to keep hungry people enslaved, give them food; if you want to free them, teach them to farm. For people wanting to expand their personal horizons, to improve their quality of life, to enhance their theatrical craft, or to learn the fundamentals of graceful movement, Samuel Avital's Body*Speak*™ Manual is the ultimate farmer's almanac.

Staying with this metaphor, I am pleased to report that my life to date, seeded and rooted in the values and ideas that Samuel helped to reveal to me at a pivotal time in my artistic development, has been a veritable garden of delights. Trained as an actor and filled with a passion for movement expression, I arrived at his studio as fertile ground, absorbing the seeds of his artistic provocations mixed with clear, simple and precise exercises. I have, over time, integrated them into virtually every aspect of my performing, directing, and teaching. I was 22 years old when I first met Samuel. And at this writing, 22 years have since passed. My life has been immeasurably enriched by my contact with this man and his work. He gave me permission to be an individual, to fall in love with the discipline and the standards of the craft; and most of all, he showed me how the truth of the body could be infinitely harvested.

While auditioning for the famed mime/mask show Mummenschanz, for example, barely two years after my first intensive with Samuel, I was asked to improvise and explore the character of several unusual mask forms. There were mime performers from all over the world at this audition, along with a number of gymnasts and established actors. I had borrowed the money to get to New York and knew that if I did not get in the show it was going to be a lean winter. My experience with masks was limited and much of that was at Samuel's studio. So, with each mask, before going on stage, I would take a long moment to focus and recollect the inner empty place I had found during the Life mask exercise in Samuel's studio. I let the truth of the body give over to the demands of the mask. Although the time I took made the stage managers uneasy, it ultimately won the day in the audition: I was one of only three hired for the international touring cast.

There are many other examples of how Samuel's teachings have influenced my life and it is no exaggeration to say that all of my work as a performer has been informed on some level by what I have learned from Samuel and his book. My process of characterization, my sense of presence, my appreciation of the organic flow of energy and the precise measure of truth, my trust in the moment-to-moment, and my commitment to playing fully at any magnitude, all owe a debt of gratitude to his teaching. In fact, I have even noticed that whenever I am doing any work for film or television, I still use the essential ingredients from Samuel's principles of Motion/Stillness.

As a director, I apply most of the principles established from his method **Body*Speak*™** on Gravity, Motion/Stillness, Leaders/Followers, Parallels, and Staccato /Slow Motion. My productions are always spatially interesting and move with dynamism reminiscent of the journeys taken in those magical classes provided by Samuel. To this day, I can hear his voice urging me to go to the edge; to have compassion for the audience and to electrify the atmosphere by tilting into the unknown.

Perhaps the greatest influence is evident in my teaching. I no longer know what part of my teaching belongs to Samuel and which part belongs to me. And in truth, it no longer matters. I belong to a long line of teachers who have all encountered the same furnace. Because I was ready and Samuel was available to me, I found myself with a movement foundation strong enough to allow me to learn Tai Chi, Alexander Technique, Stage Combat, Advanced Mime techniques and Physical Comedy in record time. I'll never forget the day that I realized that what my Alexander Technique teacher was doing was a mixture of Samuel's Standing Balance Meditation and the Snail Exercise in reverse! Once I made that connection, my work progressed geometrically. This experience was repeated in numerous variations in countless situations through the years.

His previous books, *The Mime Workbook* and *Mime & Beyond*, were a constant resource for me and for many students through the years. I used the exercises and referenced the sayings and the photos as sources of kinetic inspiration. The vocabulary of the books was instantly accessible and my own students found the work pleasurable, yet very demanding. Although more sophisticated, his newest work, ***The BodySpeak*^{TM} *Manual***, is a workbook equally accessible and inspired.

Samuel challenges us to roll up our hesitant sleeves and get to work in the creative laboratory. In his world, there are no excuses. One cannot say, "I don't have the script" or "I don't have the props" or "I don't have the space." All spaces are theatres, and the artistic resources, the producer, writer, and indeed the whole staff is within. As he calls it **"Be the Shakespeare of yourself."** He vigorously invites us to sweat, to activate, to explore, to have the courage to move in new ways, to dream, to nourish, and to do it all within the framework of very practical exercises. In ***The BodySpeak*^{TM} *Manual***, for example, Samuel introduces very valuable eye exercises with an accompanying Eye Compass chart. As Samuel knew well before Moshe Feldenkrais made it popular, the eyes are the keys to enhancing and re-patterning the kinetic nervous system.

Is it possible to integrate our finest impulses, our most noble intentions, and our truest thoughts into physical action? Is it possible that an aware body moving through space can have a profound effect on one's thinking? Can the experience of a lived moment of artistic paradox shatter the false self and bring forth a fully alive and authentic individual? Can there be unhindered access to the heart when the mind surrenders to the truth of the body?

If you plunge into the work provided within this book, you will arrive at a resounding **"Yes!"** to these and other similar questions. This book itself is a resounding **"Yes! Yes!"** to life, to courage, to honesty, to paradox, to the individual, to tradition, and even to non-traditions. Within these pages are materials of great creative force, devised and condensed over the course of a lifetime of focused, heartfelt work. Look closely and you will find directions for how to harvest and mix the materials stated in simple non-dogmatic language.

This book is a treasure trove—vibrating artifact. You cannot hold it without holding the past and future. It is connected to an invisible thread that runs back through time, through the golden ages of our greatest human cultures. When an exercise tugs on your soul, you are being touched by the past and when a phrase rings your inner gong, you are being hailed into the future. When you are true to the teachings, you are supremely here and now in a timeless flow of motion and stillness.

Move freely, but with full attention, as you make your way into the multi-layers of this marvelous book. Spend time with it, study the illustrations, read and re-read key phrases until they reveal their deeper message. Above all, do the exercises. Do them many times, alone or with others. And if you are lucky, you will one day find your self, as I did, enjoying the fruits of Samuel's teaching and perhaps planting a few seeds of your own.

Mark Olsen, January 6, 2001 Email: meo1005@aol.com - Associate Professor, Penn State School of Theatre, 124 Arts Building, Penn State University, University Park, Pa 16802

MARK OLSEN is a movement specialist, actor, director, author, and teacher. He has taught acting and movement for actors at Carnegie Mellon University, University of Houston, Cincinnati Playhouse Conservatory, and Penn State University. As a movement specialist he has choreographed and coached productions at major theatres and universities across the nation. His specialties in the movement arts include Mask-work, Mime, Alexander-based Physical Alignment, Stage Combat, Tai Chi, and Physical Comedy. In addition to his solo work, Mark has performed professionally as a leading actor with the Cincinnati Ensemble Theatre, The Human Race Theatre, and the mime/mask show Mummenschanz. He has directed over 30 productions and choreographed movement and stage fights for over 60 productions in various professional venues. Most recent examples include movement coaching for *Macbeth, Rough Crossing, Enchanted April,* and *Camino Real* at the Hartford Stage Company, *Last of the Formicans* and *The Windows of Camus* at Penn State University, *Anthony and Cleopatra, Julius Caesar, Angels in America* and *Streetcar Named Desire* at The Alley Theatre in Houston, *Pericles* at Houston Shakespeare Festival, Romeo *and Juliet* and *Carmen* at the Houston Grand Opera, and the T.V. Miniseries *Woman of Independent Means* with Tony Goldwyn and Sally Fields. Mark is the author of three books: *The Golden Buddha Changing Masks* (Gateways Press), *The Actor With a Thousand Faces,* (Applause Books) and *The Conception Mandala (Co-written with Samuel Avital, Destiny Books).* Currently based in New York, Mark continues his work as a man of the theatre in both professional and university settings.

PREFACE

DARE TO IMAGINE

by Samuel Avital

Well, here is another book for the trilogy, the *Mime Workbook* (1975), *Mime and Beyond: The Silent Outcry* (1985) and now *The* BodySpeak*TM Manual* (2001). The first two are full of images and photographs of my performances and other moments on my artistic path to discover the subtleties of human expression, plus words and exercises to assist the body to express itself totally without fear or limitations.

The BodySpeak*TM Manual* is a selection of my writings and teachings: essays, poems, stories, and new exercises for the purpose of developing kinesthetic intelligence and exploring the philosophy, theory and intention of the **Body***Speak*™ method of training. In this book there are many new exercises, in addition to those collected over the years, included in the central section called "Creative Body*Speak*™ Exercises."

In a time when fitness gyms are everywhere, I have developed the following observation...most body training is focused on defending the body, as an army does. The movements are brusque and focused solely on physical development.

The approach, probably influenced by the industrial revolution, is toward thinking of **the body as a machine**. From this perspective, the words that describe the body are re-languaged. Thus we talk of "fixing" the body, rather than "healing" it.

From another perspective, of thinking of **the body as a living organism,** I suggest throughout the exercises in this manual to gently work with the body, not with a defensive attitude, but focusing on the mental intention and breath. I have always professed that a movement that does not breathe is not a full movement.

I call this way of working with the body, **Body***Speak.*™ It is a method I have developed over the years in many workshops and with many students realizing the benefits. This work considers the body as a living organism, not as a machine.

Body*Speak*™ is a transformative art, capturing the essence of a movement through directed awareness.

Body*Speak*™ is designed for people of all professions including public speakers, actors, dancers, clowns, physicists, entrepreneurs, and people from all walks of life.

An astonishing 90 percent of what we communicate is derived from what we do rather than what we say. It is revealed in our gestures, our facial expressions, and how we use the space around us. Our nonverbal behavior must send the same message as our words; otherwise the message will be lost.

I call my school Le Centre du Silence to express the importance of silence in the art of mime and movement in general, and in particular the benefits of silence to the quality of life we live in this very noisy world.

Le Centre du Silence Mime School (LCDS) is an independent school for self-discovery through the human arts, devoted to teaching the dynamics of personal power and professional creativity. The school offers seminars and workshops that integrate thought with action by teaching theater and movement: how to learn to write your own script, play the lead role in your life story intelligently, and awaken the creative child within you, relying with confidence on your own authority.

The purpose of LCDS is to surpass the normal means of communication offered by the entertainment industry and the widespread abuse of the spoken word. The philosophy of LCDS is based on Conscious Integrated Honesty. The artistic principles taught provide you with the most honest tools of communication to relate to yourself and your environment practically and productively.

These are thoughts on silence I have shared with my students over the years and share with you now, dear reader:

Silence is not the absence of words, it is a fullness of being.

Silence as not merely the absence of sound, or noise; it is a state of being at the edge of listening to nothing…and something.

When you are in the forest and keep still, it may at first seem hushed. But as the noise in our head diminishes, we hear the forest humming, throbbing with life, and orchestrating a symphony of symbiosis. Eventually, we may even hear the background silence of our minds, wherein all of our questions arise and are resolved.

The inner space is a place where you can listen to that soft voice, a "place," not always quiet, but where silence reigns supreme.

Note to the Reader:
Traditionally, one reads a book from beginning to end. This is a valid way to learn. However, this book is designed in such a way as to be read intuitively. It is not simply information. This book may be opened and read at any point and a microcosm of the macrocosm can be discerned. It is not that one will not benefit from reading this book in an organized fashion, but that one should not be afraid to approach it intuitively. Both approaches will be rewarding. Enjoy.

And please remember, the exercises are intended to be introduced in the **Body*Speak*™** workshops and in private sessions. Feel free to try them yourself, but take care, go slowly, follow the directions carefully. And please feel free to get in touch with me if you have any questions.—Samuel

INTRODUCTION

MOVING BODY AND MIND
A NEW LOOK AT MIME

by Jane Evenson

Body*Speak*™ is difficult to place in any category. In its precise analysis of physical movement it might be described as bodywork. In its creative expressions it can look like dance. In its slow-motional meditative aspect it resembles Tai Chi. It incorporates elements of physical discipline and at the same time develops an extraordinary capacity for mental focus. But it is neither a religious practice nor a form of psychotherapy.

Body*Speak*™ is, par excellence, a method of activating creativity by activating movement — in ways that are startling, provocative, playful, exhilarating. It is made for anyone who struggles with the effects of *inertia. A*nd isn't that *all of us* from time to time? "A body at rest tends to remain at rest and a body in motion tends to remain in motion," reads Newton's law. Couch potatoes be forewarned. Body*Speak*™ is no spectator sport. The interesting thing is that its method of triggering outer movement seems to trigger an inner movement as well. *Inner* inertia, one discovers, is the real block to creativity. Body*Speak*™ overcomes the debilitating effects of this *inner*tia.

Many of its specific techniques derive from mime, yet in a whole new realization. Whereas mime is traditionally taught in a theatrical setting as a tool for honing the craft of the actor or clown, or as an art form in itself, Avital uses mime as a tool for self-discovery and for awakening creativity. "Mime is not the destination," he advises. "It's the launching platform."

"Man is the greatest mimic of all animals," said Aristotle, "and it is by mimicry that he acquires his earliest knowledge."[i] We learn by miming. At some point, though, we lose this marvelous tool of spontaneous learning, perhaps when we are taught the lesson of "Simon Says": you can only mimic Simon when he gives you permission, and if you succumb to spontaneity, you're out of the game. By these and other not-so-subtle methods, we're taught to control spontaneous expression with the check of the intellect.

"Behavior modeling," the psychological term for mimicry, became a byword in the practice of psychology in part to redress the imbalance created by hyper-analysis of behavior. But its corrective practicality is questionable when most people have lost the ability even to see what behavior they should be modeling! Or, if they do recognize the desired behavior, they are left to figure how to get their neglected and resistant bodies to reproduce it. For that matter who wants merely to imitate? As an art form, mime teaches "behavior modeling," but with a creative spin.

Avital uses the tool of mime to reawaken an elemental creative capacity. The effect can be stunning. One of his former students, storyteller Dot Ormes, gives her impression of *atelier Avital*:

Working with Samuel is somewhat like being the over-curious sorcerer's apprentice. Enticed by the deceptive simplicity of the work, I dive in and suddenly find myself drowning in a flood, with brooms marching endlessly back and forth carrying even more buckets of water to douse me. In the nick of time, the flood subsides. The Mimagician returns, grabs me by a soggy collar and we turn back to page one in the Book of Silence... .My teacher is a big ring of invisible keys — they dangle in my hands as I stand before as many unmarked invisible doors. There is no superficiality here. To slide easily on the surface of mime-form would be a betrayal of this art.[ii]

The essay "What is Body Speak?" briefly describes the framework, method, and applicability of this training. But of course the best way to acquire an appreciation of Avital's work is to experience it directly, as thousands have already done. My first acquaintance — Avital had retired briefly from teaching at the time — came through a reading of some of the essays now assembled in this collection.

I found a disarming simplicity and directness of expression that rises, frequently, to the level of poetry. The essays have the freshness of being spoken, *voix vivante*, in the workshop laboratory itself; and in fact they were for the most part dictated and then transcribed from tape recordings.

One of my particular favorites, "Facing the Mask," describes the mask session from Avital's three-week summer program. Through a series of preparatory exercises, the training reaches this climactic point. It is an occasion of perfect peace and solemnity. As I first read the account, I had an unmistakable if indefinable sense of another, subtle movement just behind the stately measure of the words. Philosophers have called it Pure Being. Poets have simply described it. I was reminded of a poem by Wallace Stevens, "The House Was Quiet and the World Was Calm," which describes the phenomenon in a literary setting.[iii]

The quiet of the house, the leaning of the reader, the merging of the reader with the calm of the surroundings, the access of perfection: there is a feeling of inner movement here as distilled in its simplicity and effect as the quiet calm that envelops the mask session. What distinguishes "Facing the Mask" as an account of such a moment, is that the narration is not an after-the-fact description of a fortuitous and transitory occurrence.

As a hallmark of the genius of Avital's method, the mask encounter is characterized precisely by its ability to elicit in the experience of the participant, and with considerable certainty of effect, the sense of attunement and wonder that it describes. All the materials have been consciously assembled for the occasion. Although individual experiences will differ in details, participants in the mask encounter describe, with remarkable consistency, an occasion of quintessential discovery whose effects continue to reverberate long after the session is concluded.

It is important in reading "Facing the Mask" to realize that it is not the script for a guided visualization in the manner that this process is normally conducted. The participants are not sitting or lying down passively with eyes closed while the narrator takes them on a meditative journey. They are active: looking at the mask, putting it on, moving around the room, then slowly and deliberately taking on various postures and attitudes as prompted by the teacher, and, finally, removing the mask to ponder it once more. The session has the aesthetic elegance and meditative feel of Japanese Noh. There are elements of visualization, but they are engaged by a fully participative *act*-or visualizing the archetypal image of Warrior or Coward, for example, and then instantaneously embodying the archetype in precise and original ways. Mark Olsen, another of Avital's former students, describes the session as "a slow, gentle handshake with the lion inside."[iv]

The approach is thus more kinesthetic than visual, but in fact all the senses must come into play and are fully integrated in service of what Avital describes as *active imagination*. Imagination becomes an animating principle: not just a manipulation of mental objects in a mental landscape, but a physical embodiment of the image or concept. The distance between thought and action is compressed in both time and space. Through a subtle dialogue of action and response, a skill is developed in these sessions that I shall call "deep orientation." Psychic space and physical space merge and one learns to navigate the mental/physical terrain. The teacher acts as a compass, pointing the way.

I am reminded of an incident in Einstein's early life, an encounter with a compass, which was to affect him deeply. The episode is related by biographer Abraham Pais:

> ...Einstein spent his earliest years in a warm and stable milieu that was also stimulating. In his late sixties he singled out one particular experience from that period: "I experienced a miracle... as a child of four or five when my father showed me a compass." It excited the boy so much that "he trembled and grew cold." "There had to be something behind objects that lay deeply hidden...the development of [our] world of thought is in a certain sense a flight away from the miraculous.v

Avital had an equally resonant experience as a child in a rendezvous with the horizon. (See "The Horizon.") On an after school adventure in his native Morocco he is lured into the countryside by the sight of a majestic tree in the distance. The young boy decides this must be the Tree of Life he has learned about in school. He concludes that the horizon line on which it stands must be the edge of the world. With sunset coming on, he reaches his destination only to discover that the edge of the world has moved and a new horizon looms in the distance! In the mist of twilight he feels embraced by the horizon and seems to merge with it. Realization comes in the words of an ancient sage: "I wandered in pursuit of my own self. I was the traveler and I am the destination."

What links these experiences is the sense of awe in an encounter with an object — a compass, a tree — that the adult world takes for granted. And both experiences are later recognized to have been, in a sense, defining moments that intimate a life direction — a compass pointing the way. Einstein never lost his sense of wonder. Avital, also, never lost the sense that something lay deeply hidden behind objects: call it the horizon, the destination, the self, the essence. Terminology is not important here. The direction might be science or art or a philosophy that links the two. What is important is the encounter itself and what is experienced and learned.

To follow the compass point, to embark on such a journey of discovery, it is necessary to begin at the beginning and look at the world with fresh eyes. For Avital that has meant the necessity to reconsider everything that we ordinarily take for granted — primary movements, sensory experience, relationship to objects and people — and to re-awaken our sense of wonder in these things, to make "the invisible, visible and the ordinary, extraordinary." In so doing, he has found a method to reproduce in the workshop laboratory an occasion for his students to experience, on multiple levels, the equivalent of Einstein's adventure with the compass or his own encounter with the horizon.

How is this accomplished? The answer may be found by retracing the route taken.

EARLY LIFE

Avital was born to a Sephardic family in the village of Sefrou near the Atlas Mountains of Morocco. He was the son of loving and hardworking parents and had a particularly close relationship with his grandfather, a respected spiritual leader of the community, successful trader, and benefactor of a charitable circle that performed its offices anonymously. It was called, with wry humor, The Society of the Lazy Ones. Avital has fond recollections of being an unwitting emissary on their secret missions of goodwill. He also recalls his grandfather's wise counsel.

On one noteworthy occasion grandfather and grandson joined in the traditional grape stomping in preparation for wine making. Up to his knees in half-fermented grapes, the boy became increasingly talkative. As was his grandfather's custom, instruction came in the gentle form of a story. Avital recounts:

"Before one is born," my grandfather said, "one is given a certain amount of words to use in one's lifetime — like a word account in a Cosmic Word Bank. You must be very careful in using words properly, and with measure, and in *how* you use them to express yourself. Every word you use is out of your cosmic account. That is why you should turn your tongue seven times within your mouth before uttering a word. Otherwise you may finish your quota early in life, and you will find yourself mute."

My grandfather's words made a very great impression on me as a young boy, no doubt contributing to my decision to make my life work in the Theater of Silence.[vi]

Community life in Morocco became a cherished memory for Avital, a remembrance of "utopia" in the root sense of that word — *nowhere*, in all his travels, again to be found. And the travels were soon to begin.

Possessed of a fierce idealism, he decided, at fourteen — above the strong objections of his family and in a dangerous time — to emigrate to Israel. It was a perilous passage. Jews were prevented by law from emigrating, and Samuel, even though traveling in disguise, was almost captured three times. He eventually reached Israel by ship and entered an entirely new phase — kibbutz life. He studied physics, agronomy, theology, art, and theater. Avital's interest in theater carried him to Jerusalem, where he met Salomon "Moni" Yakim, also destined to become a renowned teacher of mime and theater.

Another defining moment, a second encounter with the horizon, came for Avital when, in a darkened Jerusalem movie theater — a "cinema paradiso" — in front of a flickering screen, he encountered for the first time the genius of Chaplin. The film was *Limelight* and it had the effect of a revelation: movement — deft, subtle, expressive movement — was an art in itself. Movement could convey what words could not. Movement could be studied and mastered as an art form. Avital's compass began to point northwest. He talked Moni into taking the next step with him: they would go to Paris to study theater.

In Paris of the late 50's, studying dance and acting at the Sorbonne, Avital found that for the artist both misery and ecstasy were constant companions — the misery of surviving on baguettes and sardines and the ecstasy of artistic discovery. The acknowledged masters of mime — Decroux, Barrault, Marceau — introduced Avital to a vocabulary of wonders.

TEACHERS AND LESSONS

From Decroux, Avital learned the grammar of movement. He learned to analyze, minutely, the complex maneuvers of corporeal mime and then to reconstitute the analysis in movements of elegance and simplicity. Decroux's approach was scientific, detail-oriented, and supremely focused, emphasizing physical concreteness and precision of execution. He could be a severe taskmaster. Moments of humor were startling: "Samuel and Solomon," said Decroux in the midst of a session, "I see I have a prophet and a king in here." Decroux the idealist transmitted his ideals to his students: "The mime actor must have the mind of a novelist, the body of an athlete, and an ideal in his heart."[vii]

From Barrault, Avital learned the poetry of movement. Barrault was as expansive as Decroux was contained, his art as expressive as Decroux's was silent. Barrault regarded the body as the vehicle of poetry itself. Moving away from "pure mime," he endeavored to synthesize mime and text: speak like an actor, move like a mime, he said. From Barrault, Avital realized that the whole body must be the mouthpiece of expression.

Decroux the scientist, Barrault the poet. Together they had invented "subjective mime"— as distinguished from the "objective mime" of the nineteenth century.

Objective mime is primarily concerned with production of the familiar mime illusions — the invisible barrier, walking against the wind, creation of objects in space, etc. — by a system of parallels and counterweights. In the nineteenth century these illusions were enjoyed for their own sake, as an element of the spectacle of the theater. In the twentieth century, largely through the investigations of Decroux, objective mime became a means to explore the relationship between a human being and an external object or opposing force.[viii]

Subjective mime, by contrast, was an exploration of interior states: feelings, attitudes of being. Barrault defined it as the "study of states of the soul translated into bodily expression. The metaphysical attitude of the man in space."[ix] Decroux "often in his lessons spoke about how an actor carrying a heavy physical weight closely resembled one carrying a heavy metaphysical one."[x] In Avital's view, mime concretizes metaphysics. Where other arts may *represent* a concept or truth — the dancer dances it, the writer writes it, the painter paints it, the actor speaks it — the mime *becomes* it.

Drama had its origins in the sacred. Greek drama developed through the sacred arts of pantomime. By miming the actions of the gods, the gods, it was believed, were invoked and propitiated. Movement itself was a sacred principle. Heraclitus held that all was movement, flow, and change. Aristotle termed the creative principle the "Prime Mover."[x] Movement — in its infinite varying — is the basis of every created thing. As the very essence of theater, mime, in the estimation of Decroux and Barrault, was the means of returning theater to that sacred source. "In the beginning was the word. BEFORE the word there was motion, vibration, movement, the source of all life," Avital affirmed.

Through his own synthesis of the work of his great teachers, Avital realized, importantly, that as significant as the study of mime was for those with theatrical aspirations, its methods should not be sequestered in the theatrical preserve. He composed a brief fable, "The Dancing Egg" to illustrate his point. Mime, the elegantly simple, perfectly contained, dancing egg is cracked open — taken beyond its confines — to restore the past and nurture the future. The time-honored theatrical metaphor, "all the world's a stage," would finally have to be embraced in its full implications: that art and life become one. We might then achieve the condition, as in some cultures, where there is no differentiation of the two.[xi]

But part of the task of apprenticeship for anyone learning to master a skill is to apply the skill in its intended arena. For mime that arena has traditionally been the theater. Marcel Marceau, Avital's third great teacher, provided an example of applying the art to the practical realities of performance. With Decroux, performance had been out of the question: it was not allowed. Mime was reserved for the laboratory. Marceau, on the other hand, encouraged performance. "Try your wings, Samuel," he said.

Indirectly, though, Marceau's particular form of expression was to contribute to Avital's growing conviction that the techniques of mime could and should be applied beyond the theater. Like Chaplin's Tramp, Marceau's character, Bip, is an Everyman. Bip appears in every imaginable situation — Bip in the Metro, Bip the Host, Bip the Gendarme, Bip in Love, Bip Looks for a Job, Bip Commits Suicide — provoking, by turns, both pathos and mirth. Marceau's work illustrated that mime was capable of representing the gamut of human experience. So successful was his creation, though, that Marceau became its prisoner.[xii] Audiences were not receptive to Marceau outside of the character of Bip or even out of white face. Here was surely a warning of the creative hazards of theatrical performance.

As audience expectation rigidified, mime itself was to become, to a certain extent, the prisoner of Marceau's success. The silent, white-faced performance became synonymous with mime. Many who wanted to emulate Marceau's success, but who had neither his talent nor skill, donned white face and began to invade the personal space of any hapless passerby. But as Decroux, Barrault, Marceau, Avital, and also LeCoq (another renowned innovator) have demonstrated, mime is an art of great subtlety and complexity. It is not even, necessarily, a silent art. *Pantomime* is the term reserved for silent mime. *Mime*, on the other hand, may or may not be silent. It may use text or music. Silence, when it is incorporated, is like other gestures — a tool of expression.

But in the early 1960's, Marceau was just beginning to ride the crest of his fame, and through his efforts mime was gaining wider and wider recognition. Much can be learned in an encounter with an audience, and with the growing and receptive audience for mime, Avital embarked on the journeyman phase of his apprenticeship. He began to tour with Maximilien Decroux, Etienne Decroux's son, and then with his own solo show. In the meantime, Moni had left to New York. Samuel joined him there in 1964, to perform in the Pantomime Theater of New York, which Moni had founded, and in off-Broadway theaters. He also taught in New York schools.

In America, Avital felt many of the same sensations experienced by other immigrants arriving from Europe: a mixture of terror and exhilaration. America was as vast and open as Europe was tight and restricted. In America, *sans frontières*, Avital felt he could breathe and expand.

After a few years of touring North and South America, Avital was appointed artist-in-residence at Southern Methodist University (SMU). In 1971 he was invited to perform in Denver, Colorado, and decided to take a side trip to the nearby university town of Boulder. Impressed by the physical beauty of the place and by the receptivity of the people he met, Avital agreed to perform in Boulder. The day after the sold-out performance, more than 200 people showed up for Avital's first workshop. He was urged to stay and within the year had founded his own school, Le Centre du Silence. The Boulder Mime Theater was formed a year later and toured locally and nationally for nine years. In 1975, Avital established the International Summer Mime Workspace, an annual event that attracts students worldwide.

THE WORKSHOP LABORATORY

In these early years Le Centre du Silence became Avital's laboratory, where he could fully distill the teachings of the mime masters and develop his own unique methods. The work was improvisational and experimental, employing some prepared exercises along with anecdotes and stories. Students took notes and gradually the method evolved, always in direct response to the participants' needs.

Most of the students in these years came because they were interested in theater and were drawn by Avital's unique method of developing theatrical technique. But it was clear that their personal needs went beyond the requirements of professional apprenticeship. The late 60's and early 70's were a time when many people felt drawn toward deep personal and spiritual search. Avital felt concerned to develop for his students a means to engage in these explorations that would provide fulfillment but avoid some of the pitfalls of other paths that had become popular at the time.

The demands of life in the West could not be fully addressed, he understood, by methods that drew people out of the stream of life for prolonged periods. It was too easy to drop out entirely or at least to *opt* out and live life in a state of numbness, feeling personally alienated and professionally stifled. The divisions of life were taken for granted to such an extent that the task had become not only to integrate art and life but also self-discovery and life.

Creativity had always been an important issue for Avital. He found that while traditional methods might be effective in developing either physical or mental discipline, they did not directly stimulate creativity. In fact in some cases it was essential to practice the discipline *precisely* in the time-honored manner in order to realize the greatest benefit. This was true of yoga or Tai Chi or even classical ballet, and for certain types of sitting meditation practice or martial arts. Obviously great benefit can be derived through a judicious practice of these and other such disciplines. Discipline is surely the foundation of excellence in any art, including mime. It was necessary to bear in mind, though, that any discipline is not an end in itself, it is a tool of greater realization. The finger is not the moon.

Avital developed a number of exercises with the purpose of directly accessing creativity. They come into play in all the workshops but have been assembled and condensed in current format under the title, "The Journey from Thought to Action." It's an eye-opener. When Avital resumed teaching recently, I participated in this intensive weekend event.

We began with "Presentation With and Without Words." Exactly as the title of the exercise suggests, each participant is asked to introduce himself or herself first, with words, and then, without words. The second half of the exercise is followed by a group commentary, which Avital calls "The One Who . . ," with each member of the group summing up his or her dominant impression of the individual's silent presentation: The One Who Was Shy, The One Who Walked in Circles, The One Who Blew Kisses, and so on. The comments are meant to be brief and impressionistic. They have the effect of opening up the group and introducing the feedback principle: creativity does not exist in a vacuum. We are constantly taking in information, synthesizing it, and giving it back in a new form.

Another exercise, actually a series of exercises, called "Act and React," illustrated this principle in a most startling way. We began by walking around the room in a group. There were twelve of us; a comfortable size, I felt. On Avital's cue (he would strike percussion sticks together) we had to freeze in place and carry out an instruction: to represent an emotion, for example, or utter the exact thought that was in our minds the moment the sticks were clicked. The purpose was to lubricate our wheels and get us back into the practice of manifesting our thoughts with freshness and immediacy. Avital would select a few individuals to hold a pose that he found to be particularly illuminating. The rest of us would move around this living statuary, offering our own insights or marveling when someone had achieved the very essence of immobility.

Then came the magical moment. For the next activity of the exercise, we had to walk the room once again at random and then, at the instant the sticks were struck, take a pose in response to whatever occurred in our vicinity. There were no other instructions given: just act and react to each other instantaneously. We were surprised to discover that our immediate response to one another had produced a coalescence: our groupings had *meaning* as if a sculptor or director had premeditated the tableaux. The effect was as stunning as if a chemical compound had suddenly precipitated out of a solution.

For the physicist, the doctor, and the engineer who were participating in this workshop, for the lawyer who had spent her professional life wading hip-deep in language, or the 75-year-old self-declared ski-bum who wanted to try something new, or the shy woman who never dreamed she would feel so safe in such an environment, for the massage therapist, the artist, the writer, the timepiece restorer, and the professional storyteller, for the scholar who wanted her book to be true — there was something here for everyone. *"Every artistic genius is a specialized type of mime,"*[xiii] M. J. d'Udine observed after studying with Dalcroze, an innovator in the arts of movement who influenced Decroux and many others. In my weekend tour of Avital's atelier I realized the full truth of this insight.

One of the classic illusions of mime, the creation of a box in space, became "The Moving-Box Encounter." First, we learned to form the box by parallel movements of the hands. Then, we enlarged it or contracted it so that it became big enough to lean against or small enough to pop in the mouth. Next, we learned to move around the room in silence carrying and manipulating, creatively, our cube of space. Finally, we practiced transferring boxes back and forth to one another: this moving meditation had become a careful and tender, silent, *dialogue*.

The physicist had come to the workshop because he was curious about mime. "There had to be something behind objects that lay deeply hidden," said Einstein. This is a territory explored by mime that would, of course, be of interest to a physicist: *MimeWorld* where the *MimeMagician* plays with the laws of motion and sometimes upends them, defying gravity and creating objects in thin air; where *eye-knots* are tied in *superstrings*; where *MimeTime* is an arrow that bends back on itself; and *MimeSpace*, the moving box, is the original *hypercube*. Parallels, counterweights, "for every action there is an equal and opposite reaction" — physicists, engineers, and mimes are well-equipped to understand such things. And the mime embodies the knowledge.

"Apart from the five senses," Decroux wrote, "there is nevertheless one that serves the mime."[xiv] He couldn't put a name to this sense and, until quite recently, "kinesthesia" had not been given the status of being considered a "sense." It is this faculty that is activated and heightened through the explorations of mime, and that makes mime a true physics of the body, as well as an art.

THE "SIXTH SENSE"

Ever since Aristotle first identified the five senses — sight, hearing, touch, taste, and smell — we've been used to thinking that we have just these five. Because the senses can be located in clearly recognizable organs of the body — the eyes, ears, nose, tongue, skin — they are also commonly thought to be "discrete," distinct and functioning separately from one another.

Actually, the senses work in conjunction. Taste and smell, for example: food tastes bland when we have a cold. Sight and hearing reciprocate to help us judge distance and relationships between objects. Sight and touch also work together. The philosopher Merleau-Ponty describes how these two senses, once considered to operate in totally separate perceptual fields, actual coordinate. He calls this process "The Intertwining":

> The look...envelops, palpates, espouses the visible things. As though it were in a relation of pre-established harmony with them, as though it knew them before knowing them, it moves in its own way with its abrupt and imperious style, and yet the views taken are not desultory — I do not look at a chaos, but at things — so that finally one cannot say if it is the look or if it is the things that

command... We must habituate ourselves to think that every visible is cut out of the tangible, every tactile being in some manner promised to visibility, and that there is encroachment, infringement, not only between the touched and the touching, but also between the tangible and the visible... Since the same body sees and touches, visible and tangible belong to the same world. It is a marvel too little noticed that every movement of my eyes — even more, every displacement of my body — has its place in the same visible universe that I itemize and explore with them, as, conversely, every vision takes place somewhere in the tactile space. There is a double and crossed situating of the visible in the tangible and of the tangible in the visible; the two maps are complete, and yet they do not merge into one. xv

Merleau-Ponty comprehends, with great subtlety, the interrelationship of the sense of sight and of touch, but cannot quite allow that their fields could actually merge. A mime is capable of providing direct access to this knowledge — embodied knowledge — that the visual and tactile fields *do* merge, even in everyday life. We could not walk a straight line toward a destination if they didn't. In fact, the only realm in which perceptual fields are separated, artificially, is in the text of a philosopher, or in the experience of individuals influenced by that type of analysis.

Someone familiar with Avital's work might recognize in Merleau-Ponty's *chiasmus* a fair description of "The Eye-Knot" exercise. Two people stand facing each other. They make eye *contact* and visualize a cord connecting their eyes.[xvi] The goal is to move in such a way as to "tie" a knot in this cord without "breaking" it by losing eye contact. Participants typically become so absorbed that when Avital comes, stealthily, with his imaginary scissors and cuts the cord, they are startled and fall to the ground!

We do, in fact, have more than five senses. ("Five senses?" Avital asks. "What about the other 95?") And they all interrelate. Perceptual researchers have identified a number of "new" candidates for recognition as full-fledged "senses." The sense of hot or cold, for instance, is pretty basic. It is related to touch but with a thermostat attached. Pressure sensitivity is even trickier. Or how about our sense of position in space — vertical? horizontal? upside down? right side up? There is, at least, this "sixth sense" which is increasingly being recognized for the profound effect it has on the way we function as perceiving beings. This is the kinesthetic sense, or *kinesthesia*.

Kinesthesia might be termed "the common sense" because it functions to integrate the workings of the other senses. Renaissance anatomists speculated that there must be a "common sense," which coordinates the functioning of the other senses, and they attempted to locate it in various organs of the brain. We now know that organs and receptors distributed throughout the body are responsible for the kinesthetic effect.

A basic dictionary definition of kinesthesia is "the sensation of bodily position, presence, or movement resulting chiefly from stimulation of sensory nerve endings in muscles, tendons, and joints by the force of gravity."[xvii] Kinesthesia is also activated by the vestibular system, the fluid-filled organs of balance in the inner ear. In its integrative function, kinesthesia depends upon the subtle interactions of all the senses: our impressions of degrees of light and sound, visual and auditory depth perception, sense of warmth and cold and the effects of breezes — to name only a few of a multitude of sensory inputs. Kinesthesia is, in short, the sense by which we orient ourselves to the world — our internal compass.

For the mime, this sense functions in the way sight does for the painter, or taste for the gourmet cook, or touch for the sculptor, or scent for the perfumier: it is both tool of exploration and object of exploration. The purpose is to use the sense and refine it at the same time.

Martial arts expert and movement trainer George Leonard observes in *The Silent Pulse* that "This delicate, sophisticated sense...not only helps us to stand straight, but to *think* straight ... .thought is involved with the body, its balance, its ability to integrate movement and sensing and touch."[xviii]

In its full sense, kinesthesia has two aspects, **attention** and **attunement**, which arise out of the interplay of rest and motion (Avital's "Motion/Stillness" principle). *Attention* is the act of placing awareness. It is a highly conscious state depending on a clear sense of the person or thing being attended to and of one's own internal state. It is a condition of restful alertness, calm focus. When full attention is given, attunement becomes possible. *Attunement* means to come into harmony or pleasant interaction. It depends on a feeling for the natural rhythms underlying all movements — the back and forth pendulum swing of give and take. This is the sense that develops in Steven's poem, "The House Was Quiet..." and in Avital's mask session. It is this sense, also, that harmonizes the imbalance of opposites. (See "Beyond Opposites") Paradox is experienced as a "tilt" in the mind. When this tilt is played out physically, the mental tilt adjusts.

KINESTHESIA AND THE MIND/BODY SPLIT

According to psychologist Howard Gardner[xix] there are seven distinct types of intelligence: verbal, musical, logical-mathematical, visual-spatial, bodily-kinesthetic, and two types of personal intelligence — self-awareness and social skill. Gardner's scheme has been influential because it recognizes types of intelligence in addition to the verbal and logical, which have long held a privileged position in our culture.

Although there is value in making such distinctions, Gardner has acknowledged that in practice the types of intelligence cannot be precisely distinguished. They work in concert with one another to make possible such skills as eye/hand coordination. Intelligence as a whole depends on input from all the senses. Mind and body cannot really be separated from each other. The term "body-mind" has been used to point up the fact that, in effect, we think with our whole bodies.

Bodily intelligence — including full sensory awareness and attunement to body rhythms — underlies all the forms of intelligence Gardner distinguishes. Verbal and musical skill are to a great extent dependent upon a sense of rhythm, balance, and proper placement. Logical and mathematical ability also require a sense of balance and proportion. Spatial awareness and orientation are obviously kinesthetic.

Personal and social skills have an especially strong kinesthetic basis. A healthy person is described as "well-balanced." Being in harmony with others is being "in sync." Successful communication depends to a great extent on kinesthetic awareness, including a sense of speech and body rhythms and the ability to tune in to the presence of another human being. Avital recognized this principle when developing Body*Speak*™. The purpose was to activate body awareness in service of communication and to expand the communicator's repertoire, not by a simplistic reading of body language — as if it were a magically revealing secret code — but through a deep investigation of *how* the body speaks.

The kinesthetic sense is thus not really separate or isolatable from the other senses. It is enhanced by input from all the senses and must coordinate their activities. We get a feel for the presence of another by visual cues, by auditory cues, by tactile cues, and so on. This is why participants in sensory deprivation studies report losing a sense of bodily contact or presence altogether and why astronauts outside the field of gravity in the weightless conditions of space retain their self-possession and kinesthetic sense (if somewhat awkwardly).[xx]

By means of kinesthesia, each sense takes on tactile qualities. This is how a look can sometimes *feel* shockingly intimate, or words can seem to stroke — or strike. An old Chinese text has a lovely way of describing how the kinesthetic sense works: "It's like reaching for a pillow in the dark... Throughout the body are hands and eyes."[xxi]

The kinesthetic sense plays an important role in development of some of the subtler faculties. It seems to be a vital component of intuition, for example, which is often described as a "gut feeling." Explaining the source of a strong hunch, we say "I just feel it in my bones." "Presence," sometimes mistakenly equated with charisma, is another elusive concept, but it, too, is marked by a high degree of kinesthesia. Individuals with "presence" seem to fill the space around themselves.

And in its fullest sense, kinesthesia expands our understanding of the faculty of imagination. With its root term "image," imagination centers on the visual sense. Clearly, though, when we fully "imagine" something we have a complete experience of all the senses and feel kinesthetically present within that experience. It's also true that guided visualization, which has become popular in sports training as a performance enhancement technique, is much more than visual. When successfully accomplished, as in the mask session, it is a fully coordinated kinesthetic experience.

In its coordinating function, the kinesthetic sense serves to fill in from our memory bank of sense impressions whatever sensory information is missing in a message. The need to get a complete picture on the basis of limited data is a strong survival need. The gap in information is sensed as disorienting and the *active imagination* jumps in to fill it.

Our kinesthetic sense is especially active in childhood, when survival is particularly perilous. Birth is the original experience of disorientation. The *active imagination* plays a vital orientational role as the child grows and tries to make sense of a confusing world, with the kinesthetic sense contributing to a feeling of participation — of really being absorbed by an activity — that is so characteristic of childhood. The world feels alive and every pore is open to experience. We learn spontaneously, at this stage, through mimicry.

As we grow, we come to a critical period of emerging self-awareness. Visual orientation develops. We see ourselves in mirrors. We begin to regard ourselves as having distinct boundaries, as separate individuals. A gap in awareness forms: I am here...You are there. Self/Other. Some can remember their first experience of this gap. It can be a poignant memory. Inhibitions arise as we see ourselves being seen. Spontaneous mimicry ceases.

The visual sense develops further. We learn to read; we *watch* things, we watch *television*. Eventually, visual orientation can come to dominate so completely that we become obsessed with how things look. Image becomes all. The other senses lose the edge they had when we were very young and were touching and tasting everything in sight. Visually dominated, we literally "lose touch." In our hyper-visual culture, the kinesthetic sense atrophies like an unused muscle, and *too* much weight is given to visual cues. Sensory awareness must be re-awakened across the full spectrum of perceptions.

This is why mime, in Avital's world, is not a spectator sport. And perhaps why Decroux was so suspicious of performance: the uncomprehending scrutiny of an uninitiated audience was of little value to him, and, as in the case of Marceau, the act of spectating could actually distance the audience from a true perception of the function of mime, certainly as Decroux understood it. Mime in its new realization was intended as nothing less than fully co-ordinative in its functioning and fully participative in its realization.

THE RETURN TO THE BODY

In its integrative role, mime belongs in the context of a twentieth-century undertaking that we might call "The Return to the Body." The Western discovery of Eastern disciplines — yoga, Tai Chi, the martial arts — is a mark of this trend. Modern dance — as pioneered by Duncan, St. Denis, Shaw, Graham, Cunningham, and others — has sought to liberate the expressive body. Movement therapies — such as those developed by Alexander, Feldenkrais, Trager, and Rolf — have played an important role.

Psychology began to investigate the inter-relationship of mind and body. Head, a contemporary of Freud, described kinesthesia as "deep sensibility." Gestalt has brought about a complete reassessment of the nature of perception. Schilder speaks of the "body-schemes" by which we orient ourselves. A body-centered trend in psychotherapy is emerging. Somatic Psychology, a recent development that traces its origins to the early Freud and to his student Wilhelm Reich, considers that "body sensations, gestures, postures, and expressive movements are a kind of language of the unconscious."[xxii]

In the field of anthropology, Ray Birdwhistell developed "kinesics," a method of minutely analyzing communicative behavior. Edward T. Hall pioneered the science of "proxemics" in his influential studies, *The Silent Language* and *The Hidden Dimension*, which argue that gesture and use of space are a language in themselves that can vary from culture to culture.

Poets and novelists have led the vanguard of the return to the body. T. S. Eliot laments our "dissociation of sensibility." D. H. Lawrence considers the "blood knowledge" of the body and "reciprocity of touch" to be the only real hope for human redemption. Poet Theodore Roethke sings sensual praise of "a woman lovely in her bones."

Popular writers have taken up the chorus. Diane Ackerman saturates us with *A Natural History of the Senses*. Morris Berman writes eloquently and urgently of the need for *Coming to Our Senses*. Michael Murphy has recently produced an encyclopedic assessment he calls *The Future of the Body*.

Philosophy in this century has at last begun to address the full implications of the Cartesian legacy of mind/body dualism. The subtle analyses of Merleau-Ponty and the highly original reflections of Gaston Bachelard represent the pinnacle of this endeavor.

All of these efforts, and this is of course only a selective inventory, have played a part in correcting the imbalance created by a host of "isms" — including Puritanism, Romanticism, Victorianism, as well as various strains of philosophic Idealism and religious mysticism or gnosticism — that had discredited or denied the body, or upheld an otherworldly ideal in which the body played at best a marginal role. Twentieth century human beings arrived at the supposed final "ism," the Deconstructionism of the 1970's, with nowhere else to go.

Morris Berman calls this tragic tale of flight from the body "the hidden history of the West" and makes his own plea for reunion. Yet Berman himself admits, in his candid epilogue to *Coming to Our Senses*: "This has been a difficult book for me to write; I struggled a lot with my own body, which I love and hate, as the pages were filling with ink." He wonders if he may in fact have "overvalued the body as a vehicle of cultural integrity":

> We can recognize the tremendous drawback of the mind/body split, and the severe limits of dualism and a dualistic culture; but body integrity finally doesn't necessarily get you into the social or natural environment, and there is no way that these can be ignored.[xxiii]

If Berman struggles in a love/hate relationship with his own body, he may not truly know whether body integrity, fully realized, can "get you into the social or natural environment." He regrets:

> Something obvious keeps eluding our civilization, something that involves a reciprocal relationship between nature and psyche, and that we are going to have to grasp if we are to survive as a species. But it hasn't come together yet, and as a result, to use the traditional labels, it is still unclear whether we are entering a new Dark Age or a new Renaissance.xxiv

Berman is surely correct in observing that "it hasn't come together yet," in spite of the dedicated efforts of the artists, psychologists, and philosophers mentioned in our brief survey. Pioneer visionaries do not any longer have the option of retiring to a basement atelier with Decroux or to the woods of Maine with Thoreau — who had longings of his own:

> I stand in awe of my body, this matter to which I am bound has become so strange to me. I fear not spirits, ghosts, of which I am one...but I fear bodies, I tremble to meet them. What is this Titan that has possession of me? Talk of mysteries!—Think of our life in nature,—daily to be shown matter, to come in contact with it.,—rocks, trees, wind on our cheeks! the solid earth! the actual world! the common sense! Contact! Contact! Who are we? where are we?xxv

Thoreau wails where Berman sighs, but the same concern haunts both: where have we arrived in our headlong technological rush? can we much longer endure the divisive legacy of our systems of thought and belief? how do we redeem the natural world and a community that has lost its way? In partial response, Berman cites Decroux, who once remarked "that people should walk down the street as if they belonged to each other."xxvi More is required, of course, but we might also cite Barrault, who speaks very differently from Thoreau:

> Life has been given to us? A great thanks! I will never do enough to be worthy of this gift. Modern society, carried today in a sort of toboggan of destruction, can leave me lost and wandering in the middle of a pile of ruins; that doesn't bother me anymore. In giving me life one made me: a body. An integrated body, a magnetic body which, giving me the universe for parents, tells me what I have to do: to connect myself with it.

> This body which I love as much as I love life, I must be worthy of. I am at the same time astonished and marveling... . I am not against anyone. I am ready, on the contrary, to bring my humble share to the community.xxvii

Apocalypticism may be just too grandiose a mood to be indulged any longer. We already know that the Emerald City is an overrated destination and that "there's no place like home." How do we get there? The answer, Avital would say, is right under our noses.

Melissa Huntress, a long-distance runner who took Avital's three-week summer program and is currently working privately with him, speaks about the effect of the training.xxviii Each physical improvement has been accompanied by another change that is even more subtle and meaningful. Practice of Avital's exercise cycles enables her to lift out of her pelvis and breathe more fully; her motion "is more directed and organized" and she runs "with less effort." She is also "beginning to feel or sense a very subtle internal circular movement of energy — an ebbing and flowing, a rising and falling." At the same time she notices that she is more able to feel her own source of power and motion. She calls the experience a feeling of "deeper will." "Best of all," she says, "*I* make the decision to be running this way now. Before I would have this experience randomly or accidentally."

But another phenomenon is occurring, one that might interest both Berman and Thoreau. By practicing Avital's perceptual exercises she experiences increased depth and dimension of perception, as if she is fully embracing, with all her senses simultaneously, the terrain through which she runs. She has a feeling that she is no longer just running past scenery: "I am now able to draw on the power of things I am running by." She is very careful to explain that her experience of this is something much more focused and intelligible than "runner's high." Perhaps it is the "elusive obvious" that Berman mentions: "something that involves a reciprocal relationship between nature and psyche, and that we are going to have to grasp if we are to survive as a species."

He says this relationship "hasn't come together yet," but evidently there is a way it can: a method that is a physics of the body as well as an art form, that unites aesthetic cultivation and physical discipline, that integrates body and mind in service of imagination and creativity, that activates deep sensibility and a deeper will and permits nature and psyche to link up on a morning run — a body-mind compass known as Body*Speak*™.

Boulder, Colorado January 2001

JANE EVENSON has degrees in philosophy and literature. She works as a business consultant to support her explorations of kinesthetic intelligence. She has known Samuel Avital and admired his work for over nine years.

NOTES TO THE INTRODUCTION

i   Comprising essays and shorter reflections from *Mime Workbook* (Wilmot, WI: Lotus Light Publications, 1982) and *Mime and Beyond* (Prescott Valley, AZ: Hohm Press, 1985) as well as selected unpublished essays, stories, and the autobiographical sketch "The Horizon." All quotations from Avital are from these works or from private conversations unless otherwise noted.

ii   *Poetics:* IV, 2. Quoted in Marcel Jousse, *The Oral Style*, trans. Edgard Sienaert and Richard Whitaker (New York: Garland Publishing, 1990) 24.

iii   *Mime and Beyond*, 103.

iv   In this introduction, *phenomenon* is used in the philosophical sense of perceptual event or occurrence.

v   Wallace Stevens, *The Collected Poems of Wallace Stevens* (New York: Alfred A. Knopf, 1975) 358-9.

vi   *Mime and Beyond*, 101. Mark Olsen, a theater professor and former Mummenschanz performer, is also author, along with Avital, of *The Conception Mandala*, a guide to techniques of conscious conception.

vii   *"Subtle is the Lord": The Science and the Life of Albert Einstein* (New York: Oxford University Press, 1982) 37.

viii   From an unpublished manuscript.

ix   Avital's personal recollection of Decroux's frequently recited dictum.

x   Thomas Leabhart, *Modern and Post-Modern Mime* (New York: St. Martin's Press, 1989) 62.

xi   Quoted in *Modern and Post-Modern Mime*, 63.

xii   *Modern and Post-Modern Mime*, 64.

xiii   Leabhart notes that in Bali art and life are so well integrated that there is "no separate word for art." *Modern and Post-Modern Mime*, 126. See also "Hands," p. 42 of this collection.

xiv   "I am a prisoner of my art. People do not want to see me speak, or use props or appear as a character other than Bip or the stylized mime that I have created. They are uneasy with a Marceau that is unfamiliar." Quoted in *Mime and Post-Modern Mime*, 75.

xv   Quoted in *The Oral Style*. p. 24.

xvi   Etienne Decroux, *Words on Mime*, trans. Mark Piper (Claremont, CA: *Mime Journal*, 1985) 81.

xvii   Maurice Merleau-Ponty, *The Visible and the Invisible* (Evanston: Northwestern University Press, 1968) 133-4.

xviii   Compare with these lines from "The Exstasie" by poet John Donne: "Our eye-beames twisted, and did thred/ Our eyes, upon one double string;/ So to'entergraft our hands..." Renaissance anatomists theorized that sight was caused by a beam which was emitted from the eye and touched the object seen.

xix   *The American Heritage Dictionary* (Boston: Houghton Mifflin, 1980)

xx   George Leonard, *The Silent Pulse* (New York: Arkana, 1986) 44.

xxi   Howard Gardner, *Frames of Mind* (New York: Basic Books, 1985).

xxii   In the early 70's, Avital was asked to train a group of astronauts to experience "weightlessness" on earth in preparation for "moon-walking" in space. (The moonwalk is a classic technique of illusionistic mime.)

xxiii   Thomas and J. C. Cleary, trans. *Blue Cliff Record*, vol. 3 (Boulder: Shambhala Publications, 1977) 571. My rendering of a slightly longer text.

xxiv   Juliet Wittman, "Somatic Psychology: Taking Your Body to Therapy," *Nexus* (Sept/Oct 1993) 20.

xxv   Morris Berman, *Coming to Our Senses* (New York: Bantam Books, 1990) 343-4.

xxvi   Henry David Thoreau, *The Illustrated Maine Woods*. ed. Joseph J. Moldenhauer (Princeton: Princeton University Press, 1974) 71.

xxvii   *Coming to Our Senses*, 344.

xxviii   Ibid., 344.

xxix   From "Le Langage du Corps," transcription of a lecture given by Jean-Louis Barrault, June 2, 1980, at Zellerbach Playhouse.

xxx   From workshop notes and private conversations.

E S S A Y S

Transcribed from teaching sessions

These articles were written as teaching tools,
delivered as workshops and public lectures with audience participation,
along with exercises to demonstrate the practical and experiential aspects
of the philosophy of the **Body*Speak*™** method.

EXPERIENCE OF A YOUNG MIME *

It is as a student in Fania Luvitch's Course in Dramatic Art that I had the experience of working with the engaging exercises of the Stanislavsky method. Though the students had a choice, during these improvisation exercises, of silent or spoken expression, for me personally no "word" was necessary. One particularly striking example illustrates what I mean. In one of theses classes, we were given the following improvisation exercise: we had to develop a scene in which we outwardly expressed the feelings of greatness and smallness. Our teacher's instruction still sounds in my ears, just as it was given to me before my improvisation: "*Accept* being small, *accept* being great..." and I ACCEPTED. The great influence of this word "*Accept*" has followed me to this day.

To develop myself toward the horizons to which I am drawn in the Dramatic Art, I also learned dance. My purpose was to have a bodily experience of the stage along with my textual studies and the course exercises and improvisations. While performing in the Jerusalem Theatre (in Israel), a Hebrew speaking theatre, I was attracted to the beauty of the French language that would, in the future, enable me to continue my studies in France. But at the same time, I observed that the value of words had started to become less necessary to my artistic expression, and I devoted myself more to the realm of gesture and bodywork. Finally, I decided to turn completely to acting without words. But I was only an amateur, and wanting to perfect myself in the Art of Mime, I came Paris to study in the School of Etienne Decroux.

With Etienne Decroux, we studied the ABC of the human body and, what is called, body grammar and diction, along with exercises that were difficult for me to perform—because my morphology did not enable me to achieve immediate mastery of my body, but through which I now have attained a moderate and meaningful degree of accomplishment.

With his wisdom and his psychological understanding so uplifting to the student, Etienne Decroux knew how to make his disciples enter fully into this study of Mime of which he my first teacher. Questions were beside the point in his classes because his explications were sufficient so as to include them all. I learned that the human body, being only a living structure, must—like a field furrowed and sown—be guided and worked in its theatrical expression, without servitude to the spoken word. To do this it was necessary, first, to submit oneself to the discipline of the exercises that in the end became a source of pleasure; second, to achieve the clarity and precision of gesture or *realized* movement; third, to possess the bodily mastery that assures a confident presence on stage.

I felt the loss of my teacher after his departure for the United States in 1959, and joined the Mime class of Marcel Marceau in order to continue my studies.

At the same time I began to study with Maximilien Decroux, who especially believed in ensemble Mime. The artistic maturity and the theatrical experience of Mime that I possess today are due to the concrete, daily work of these last two years (1959-1960) with him. Maximilien's working method developed my own personality and opened me to new horizons that I believe must guide me in the way that is my future. His teaching was given with the purpose of developing the student's personality—if it exists, and I owe to his direction what progress that I was able to make while in his company. I had the opportunity to be a member of his Mime Company, and this involvement greatly enriched my experience.

Through these personal experiences, I arrived at the following conclusions: The discipline of Mime must be all-encompassing and with right intention; it must have an exact and immediate understanding of what needs to be expressed, and at the same time translate it through the language of gesture and bodily expression.

Samuel Avital

I will not elaborate here either on the subject of body mastery that the mime must possess before all, which gives the student the possibility of developing a personal ease, style and aesthetic manner on stage, or on the subject of mastery of the mind, which enables the mime to control and direct his thought with exactness on a given theme. These two masteries provide the means for expressing and externalizing a feeling of directly transmitting thought by gesture, comprising what is called the "Act" or "Acting".

To have practiced Mime daily with love is in itself a drama. It is this drama, which has become a personal one through the course of my work, which gives me the strength to believe in a better future for the art of Mime as an autonomous and exact and self-sufficient Art.

**"One is what one is and what one becomes with intentionally
directed will and with implacability."**

(Quoted from **Souvenirs et Notes de Travail d'un Acteur [Memories and Working Notes of an Actor]**, by Charles Dullin, Paris: O. Lieutier, 1956, page 85.)

* **Experience d'un Jeune Mime**," – Written by Samuel Avital in February 10, 1961, — *Essay first published in* **Art et Danse**, *Paris, France, Sept.-Oct., 1961*. Translated from the French into English by Robert G. Margolis, Sunday, December 24, 2000.

WHAT IS BODY*SPEAK*™?

Using the art of movement as medium and metaphor, Body*Speak*™ is an interactive and highly intensive program of training designed to integrate mind, body, and spirit. It is the culmination of my thirty years experience as a theatrical performer, author, and teacher.

Body*Speak*™ is, in its essence, a journey from thought to action. Along the way we learn to focus the mind, discipline the body, and activate powerful creative energies. We discover new and subtle ways to communicate with one another. We also have a lot of fun.

THREE PHASES OF UNDERSTANDING

Body*Speak*™ training proceeds through three basic phases of understanding
— and the process of creativity:

MENTAL

We explore the intellectual and philosophical basis of the training. Our objective is to overcome a limited mindset and decode the symbols of our mental maps.

PHYSICAL

We examine the nature of corporeal experience, revealing physical and emotional characteristics through specific exercises.

INTEGRATIONAL

We combine and apply the principles studied in phases one and two by performing improvisationally in group sessions.

Phase 1	Phase 2	Phase 3
Mental/Abstract	**Physical/Concrete**	**Integrational**
Concept/Intellect	**Structure/Form**	**Application/Create**
Image/Invisible	**Manifesting/Visible**	**Completion/Existence**
Stillness/Immobility	**Movement/Dynamic**	**Building/Becoming**
Thinking Field	**Acting/Doing/Corporeal**	**Producing/Being**

FORMATS

The Body*Speak*™ training is generally conducted in different formats: a 10-week series of once-a-week evening sessions that permits an "interval training" effect; weekend thematic intensives which compresses time and space and trigger multiple "eureka" moments; a 5-day intensive that permits an even more in-depth exploration of a theme; and our climactic event, now in its 30th season, the annual International Summer Mime Workspace, which in a 3-week framework thoroughly develops all ten essential components of Body*Speak*™.

THE TEN ESSENTIAL COMPONENTS

Body*Speak*™ developed out my experience performing, and training others to perform, the time-honored art of mime. I discovered that the practice of mime demanded a unique mental and physical discipline that could be transferred to everyday life, and with rich rewards.

Mime, I recognized, was a kind of *moving meditation*. It provided the practical benefits of sitting meditation — relaxation, improved focus and concentration, self-discipline, mind-body integration — in the context of movement. Since everyday life provides far more opportunities for activity than for sitting still, the benefits seemed clear.

Through mime I also discovered a method of mind-body integration that truly activated individual creativity, that provided a vehicle for the creative energies naturally generated when mind, body, and spirit work in unison. Body*Speak*™ is firmly grounded in principles of *artistic* expression.

Finally, it was very important to me that the method I developed would provide a means not only for creative expression, but also for *authentic* expression. It had to enhance feelings of individuality, responsibility, personal freedom and power. It had to make honest communication possible. Here again the theatrical metaphor came into play: the world is a stage, we are players, we play roles, we wear masks. The question becomes: "How do we learn to play our roles competently, authentically, and responsibly?" The mask, one of the Ten Essential Components of the Body*Speak*™ method, became a dynamic tool for developing the sense of personal presence, authenticity, and power.

Since the objective of Body*Speak*™ is mind-body integration, I knew that the method itself had to be fully conceptualized and thoroughly integrated. Thus the Ten Essential Components are presented in such a way that each component builds on that which precedes it:

1. MOTION/STILLNESS

Is an exploration of the two states that compose the basis of human activity. Inner images are manifested outward in action. Breathing is balanced to activate physical and mental alertness.

2. THE EDGE

Develops an understanding of the law of gravity within the body, and demonstrates how to use this force creatively in performance and life situations.

3. BASES/FOUNDATION

Proposes to treat the human body as an architectural form, grounded and harmonious. It makes possible an untraditional way of thinking with the whole body.

4. FIXATIONS

Breaks down large movements into small physical movements. The purpose is to rediscover the whole and find out how the whole is made. It then becomes possible to fix one part of the body in space, develop the attention to details in space, and move the rest of the body around that center-point, as centre-fixé. Mastery of this principle develops clarity and precision of movement, creating different points of reference on different geometrical planes.

5. ISOLATION/UNDULATION

Are two basic rhythms explored first by teaching the body to move one part at a time with sharp, isolated movements. The isolated movements are then integrated to produce the rhythm of undulation. Upon integrating these rhythms mentally and physically, the participants experience as never before a sense of balance and well being.

6. THE SNAIL

Provides a subtle experience of touch through close observation of the movement of the snail. The approach and withdrawal techniques of the snail reveal a rhythm, both quick and slow, embodying both caution and gentleness of touch.

7. PARALLELS

Studies the way body movements mirror one another. Any movement of one part of the body has a parallel in another part, whether or not we are aware of it. This geometrical study of movement is developed through the concept of counterweight — equal and opposite forces in motion. When the body learns the vertical, horizontal, diagonal, spiral, and circular movements, the process of vertical/lateral thinking is enhanced. Thoughts and actions are then integrated more consciously, consistently, and naturally.

8. LEADERS/FOLLOWERS

Reveals the benefits, limitations, and potentials of leading and following by assigning different parts of the body to play the different roles. Harmony is achieved by the proper functioning of each part in a balanced response of activity and passivity.

9. ANIMALS/ELEMENTS

Studies the natural states of animals and elements in order to teach the body immediate response and alertness. The goal is to appreciate the gift of consciousness, and to avoid being dependent. When the body plays elements or animals — stiff as wood, alert as a cat, fluid as water, still as a mountain — a tremendous power hidden within the self is discovered which sharpens awareness in thought and action.

10. MASKS AND STICKS
- the ultimate tools of self discovery.

Masks dramatically unleash the power of personal honesty in making conscious, intelligent choices. The strategy is to develop keen observational skills; the objective is to identify reality without the influence of deceiving external "voices"; the goal is for the individual to become the author, producer, and lead actor of his or her own life.

The participants make their own masks, experience how masks solve problems, and use them to explore the phenomenon of artistic presence and to reach the essence of their natural independent self.

Sticks are the ultimate object, the metaphorical vertical/horizontal object—both archetypal and concrete. They realign physical/mental integrity and activate a dynamic principle of creativity. With the sticks playing a variety of roles—violin, broom, pencil, prison bar, fan, fishing rod, table, door — the participants improvise individually and in group application. One stick can create a whole environment and countless comical situations.

Stick-play sharpens awareness and alertness and demands 100% presence. "The Stick Circular Discipline," and "On Your Toes" awaken the group to readiness, playfulness, and creativity. The group members discover new dimensions of relating to the body, the self, and others, in ways they never thought possible. This is learning through laughter.

Throughout the training, numerous additional and complementary exercises are introduced — 75/25, the Great Puzzle, Hand-and-Foot Work, the Posture of Enchantment, The Geometry of Motion, and many others — which enrich and stimulate the creative efforts of the group.

The participants will learn to practice daily "The Longevity Cycles," a powerfully integrative series of essential exercises which enhance the effectiveness of the Body*Speak*™ training. The Longevity Cycles are comprised of:

1. THE FLEXIBILITY CYCLE (1)
is designed to gently limber and focus all parts of the body and

2. THE REGENERATIVE CYCLE (2)
integrates physical, mental and emotional attention to lubricate and
regenerate the entire organism and

3. THE INTEGRATIVE CYCLE (3)
is a profound sequence to balance and focus your life force and theatrical skills.

4. THE SELF-EVOLUTION CYCLE (4)
is a practical series of ten (10) exercises to better your life, develop your
balanced self-guidance, and quicken your personal evolution.

THE ULTIMATE JOURNEY

Body*Speak*™ workshops are a potent and adventurous journey to discover and apply your inner power, to achieve in a short time what others take a lifetime to realize. Dare to take this adventurous journey...

from **Thought** to **Word** to **Action**

from **Idea** to **Image** to **Product**

from **Chaos** and **Confusion** to **Order** and **Balance**

from **Weakness** to **Power**

from **Limitation** of **Thought** to **Freedom** of **Movement**

from **Mediocrity** of **Mere Existence** to **Excellence** of **Living** and **Being**
from **Sleepwalking** to **Conscious Awakening**

THE GOAL

The goal of the Body*Speak*™ method is quite simply to improve the quality of life of all who participate. I have had many opportunities for joy and satisfaction over the years to learn from participants in the training that they have gained new insight, sharpened their awareness and sensitivity, improved their ability to express and communicate an idea, and in many cases have changed the course of their lives as a result of their participation in the workshops. After three rewarding decades, our work at Le Centre du Silence continues.

PRACTICAL HAPPINESS

My Journey from Thought to Action
A brief account of my Parisian times

Through the study of mime, I learned to integrate creative techniques from theater, dance, music, and writing into a single productive and functional unit. Standard practice in the theater is that separate individuals perform different tasks: an author writes a play, the director directs it, the actors interpret it, the composer composes the score, and the dancer dances it.

While studying in Paris with Etienne Decroux, Marcel Marceau and Jean-Louis-Barrault, I discovered that in mime there are no authors to write the scripts. I had to be my own author, actor, director, and composer. This proved to be a challenging effort. I had to integrate all of these specializations and become my own complete mini-theater.

As I developed my craft, I experienced a sense of elation in being able to use all of my abilities. I guided myself without depending on the written words of another author and without speaking words that were not of my own creation. I became the instrument of my inner voice. By directing my creations myself, I was the one who had to see the crucial details and the total vision simultaneously. To interpret the vision with integrity, my own philosophy had to be well integrated.

To think one thing and to do another, in essence to split the expressions, is very dangerous because it creates conflicts and problems where they should not exist. I had to eliminate this conflict or risk becoming creatively stagnant. In the silence of a mime performance, the audience can readily sense this dichotomy.

My belief is that human beings naturally desire to behave honestly in thought and action. The life struggle sometimes gets in the way, however, and the mind devises deceptive survival strategies. But the body retains its innocence and reveals the deception by subtle indications. The conflict, between mind and body is eliminated when the two work together.

In mime performance, the conflict is sometimes resolved by introducing the value of "heightening" or contrast: the body slouches, head hangs low, the face grins absurdly. The audience recognizes the disparity and laughs. Humorous contrast or amplification can have the same effect in everyday life, resolving conflict and dispelling tension.

In my career I have met many thinkers who think and doers who do, but in a very fragmented manner. It is as if there is a junk shop with a merchant who has apparently unrelated items to sell. An integrated thinker walks into the shop, asks for nails, leather, glue, cloth, hammer...and produces a pair of shoes.

Non-integration and the splitting between mind and body are rampant in our society. The condition develops when people lack the confidence to think for themselves and then rely on guidance and approval from external authorities in order to function. The splitting between mind and body happens automatically when someone tries to behave according to a script written by someone else.

This is precisely why the discipline of mime became for me such an invaluable practice. Writing my own script became routine! I had to eradicate every inclination to laziness or dishonesty on the spot, making no compromises. My sense of responsibility increased in proportion to my passion for living. I became more decisive, closing the gap between thought and action. My art became one with my life. I achieved a state which may best be described as practical happiness. I then attempted to show others how they could achieve the same fulfillment.

COMMUNICATING
WITH THE BODY*

Mime uses silence and the body as tools for communication. When you write a book you take some consonants, some vowels, some commas and other writing materials and put them together in a certain way, according to your understanding, so that they express your thought fully. Eventually you have a book. It is the same idea with the body. Mime is a tool for self-discovery. With it the body can express itself. Bodies are letters in constant motion. Start with one movement, add another, and eventually you have a whole piece.

The techniques of mime help to integrate mind and body. Harmony of mind develops through using the imagination and becoming aware of the movements, actions, and reactions used in presenting oneself. When the muscles and breathing are truly moving in tune with the mind, the psyche is free to experience the meaning of subject and object, time, space, and consciousness.

Bodies are like broken vessels; they have to come together. Before this can happen you must know the shape of every piece and how it relates to the other pieces around it. Every area of the body has its own being. In order for the whole body to do one perfect movement with no broken pieces, first take it apart piece by piece. See what each part is made of. Learn how each part moves and teach it new techniques of movement. Decompose in order to recompose later. When we say decompose, we mean it in its essential sense — to de-compose, to examine the particles that form the composition.

The key is *attention*, not *tension*. Teach the different body areas to relax before they act. Whenever you make a movement, be occupied with it. Do it consciously. Concentrate, focus on it. Become "pregnant" with what you are learning. Then something will be born.

Concentration doesn't take any effort; it is effortless. Just be with whatever part of the body or whatever thought or project you are working on. You never need to *try* to do anything. Just *DO* it! Express effort without effort. In mime, you can push a 10-ton truck uphill all by yourself. If you exert the energy it would really take, you would be exhausted by the time you were finished. Instead, when each body part knows what its own individual movement is, the whole action can take place easily and appear intensely real. Give - the - place - and - time - to - every – move – ment.

Mistakes are fine as long as you correct them. As soon as you see a mistake, correct it immediately. When you notice the pelvis is not in the right place, simply send a telegram to that body part. Mistakes are our teachers. Find out which areas of the body do not listen and teach them to listen. Find out which areas of the psyche don't listen, and do the same thing. Every situation teaches something if we know how to listen for it.

Stay within your own possibilities. Do what *you* can do. If you're sloppy, so what? Know that you're sloppy and learn to be more precise. If you're precise, good. Learn more precision. In order to prevent accidents in any movement, be lucid, awake, alert. Awareness prevents accidents.

---

* Adapted from "Archetypes in Mime," *Mime and Beyond.* 40-1.

The movements open the doors to perfection and the unknown. After perfecting a technique, forget about it. After you give up a technique, you can *become* it. It will be embodied in all of your movements and actions.

It is not enough to learn decomposition in body parts, exploring them and mastering their movements. You must *remember* to do them once you know them. The word remember has two parts: *re* and *member*. That means putting the different members of the body back together after they have been taken apart. After dismembering comes the reassembling. All the pieces of the broken vessel come together, but now they are equipped to fulfill their purpose and potential as a vessel. Assembling all the parts means looking at the whole picture.

There is more to creating a mime piece than knowing isolated movements. As was said before, they must be combined in a certain way according to your understanding so they express your thought fully. A nice body making precise movements is not enough.

But just as you learn grammar so thoroughly that you forget it by the time you write a fully expressive book, so do you discover physically all the laws of movement before the body can finally express itself fully. The scientific aspect of the artist is to put the fragments in a frame. When you have reached that place, you will be able to walk through the door marked "Unknown."

ARTISTIC ZERO*

Everything that happens at Le Centre du Silence is done to bring about radical changes in our *ways of thinking*. Many people think in words, but few think in movement and vision. Learn to think in images as well as words. Every moment is a new moment. We cannot hold onto the thought or image of a moment ago because this is a brand new moment.

Nothing that happens at Le Centre du Silence is accidental. This is true in terms of both *what* is said and done and the *way* in which it takes place. A teacher is a reminder. If he speaks harshly, there is a purpose for it. He must hint, but he shouldn't point the way. Otherwise, he stifles the imagination. A true teacher provides a nourishing environment in which the imagination may flourish.

Each of us comes to Le Centre du Silence ready to learn about the integration of words and images. We eat the creative food that is offered according to our hunger.

When people come together they carry with them thoughts, fears and personal histories. A person shouldn't write on paper that already has writing on it. The paper must first be erased. There is much that we must unlearn. On a blank, fresh sheet, a person can write anew.

The body will not often listen to what it is told to do. Comfortable, secure habits keep us from giving time and space to something new. What makes you resist receiving? "I'm used to it," you say. If you are heading for a fall and your ego gets involved in trying to stop you, you will get hurt. If you relax instead, the body will take care of itself. Sometimes, the ego is out of place. Keep the ego from getting involved when it is not needed.

The body can be occupied with only one thing at a time. Any thought distracts. For example, the thought of panic causes the body to panic. Without that thought, the body would simply obey other commands. We are always afraid of breaking our bones or hurting our egos. By not trusting our bodies, we allow fear to be in us. When there is no thought of fear, there is no fear. When you find out what you are afraid of, fear can be released.

There is a plumb line that passes through the top of the skull, down the spine, through the just-kissing heels, and on down into the center of the earth. In "artistic zero," we stand sensing this imaginary line, breathing normally, eyes focused beyond the horizon. The caravan of thoughts goes by, but we pay no attention to it. In "artistic zero," we do nothing at all. It is a standing meditation and the origin of all movement — the place of still, empty listening.

Even when standing still and empty in zero, there is always movement in the body. If you let this movement take your weight in any direction, you will reach a point beyond which you will fall. This is an important place. It is your limit, your edge.

Each and every person is limited in many ways. Only when you know your limits will you know what it means to go beyond them. When you go beyond your limits, you can discover the unlimited. Limitations are doors to the unknown. Learn to know them intimately.

---

* Adapted from "Archetypes in Mime," *Mime and Beyond.* 40-1.

Stand in "artistic zero" and lean until you reach your edge. Now lean further still...Discover what is beyond the limit...A single step! That's all! That step stops the fall. The step is the beginning of something new — the next movement.

Beyond the limit is the land of the unknown. Don't be afraid of it; fear is just a limit like any other. When you go beyond fear, there is a sudden calm. When you go into the unknown, it disappears because you have filled it. Before taking the next step always find "artistic zero," even if it's only for an instant. That which has an end is subject to gravity. That which has no end is not. The unknown is endless, but there will always be a step, an image, or an idea to stop the fall if we trust "artistic zero."

The way you ask a question determines how you find the answer. Learn to ask the question with your whole body. See with your pelvis. Smell with your eyes. Swallow with your nose. To perceive the ideas that lie in the world outside our minds, we must seek total lucidity.

Life is a study of illusions. Mime seeks to insert some truth into the illusions by reflecting them. When you are in the land of the unknown and an image comes to you, let it occupy you completely. The image must be clear in every detail before the body can reflect it. It is not enough if it is just a feeling. Behind every movement there must be clarity. Then, expression occurs.

The right time to begin anything is when there is silence. The right time to act, move or speak is when there is silence. We must place ourselves in a receptive state. If we forget, the teacher is there to remind us. The intention is to release fear. We are working for total lucidity and for freedom of the imagination.

ARCHETYPAL MOVEMENT *

Theatrical activity is a necessity for a community. It is the responsibility of the artist or performer to keep that necessity alive. In storytelling, the mind of the audience must be kept right there, expectant, hanging on to every word. Stop the sentence in the middle, and the audience fills in the blank. When an audience feels that, minds can't wander. This same feeling must be transformed into performing mime. The audience must be part of the performance. It must be transfixed, eagerly awaiting the next gesture.

Every mime piece has a skeleton, flesh, and skin. The skeleton is abstract. The flesh is concrete. The skeleton is the story line. The flesh is the movement, and the skin is the quality of the execution. How can we get that quality of execution that makes an audience actually *live* the experience of watching the performance?

There are many kinds of matter. Each has an essence. Each has an archetype. By holding the image of the substance clearly in mind, we can let our bodies become the essence of the matter physically.

When a mime drinks a cup of water, it is the cup of the cup of the cup. It is the archetype of cup or container. It should be the original cup of water that the first human being drank. That cup is a blend of the specific and the general. One must sift through lots of specifics to find the general. In mime, you reach the cause, the *essence* of a situation. You must be neither too specific nor too abstract.

A mime never sips 1963 French Pinot Noir from a blue crystal champagne glass. There is no label on the bottle of a mime. He sips wine from a glass. He shows us the *essence* of wine by its effect on his nose, tongue, and equilibrium. He shows us the *archetype* of the wine glass by its delicacy, shape, and fragility. The mime must also seek essence in situations. He is not the Lone Ranger riding Silver, but a cowboy on a horse. If a mime piece is to be understood immediately anywhere in the world it must not be cultural, but archetypical in all respects.

For instance, how can the body be wood? How can the *whole* body absorb the thought of wood and express it without *acting* it? Wood has definite characteristics. It has rigidity and a certain texture. But what is the archetype? Take the pure image of wood and let the body wear it like a cloak. Suppose the wood thinks. How would it walk? Don't think just with the foot or just with the leg. Think with the whole body. The body itself must become wooden.

There are many kinds of matter: stone, wire, water, melting wax, freezing icicles, clay, feathers, vegetables, rubber, mercury. Each has an essence. Each has an archetype. By holding the image of the substance clearly in mind, we can let our bodies *become* the essence of the matter physically. *Be* clay. Melt like a burning candle. Be sincere with the image. After the body learns the essence of a substance, it can apply it to a character. Become a "wooden" person, a "rubbery" man, a "watery" woman or a "wiry" cat burglar. Each has its own integrity of movement. No matter what events befall the character, the essence is retained.

The same technique of "wearing the image like a cloak" can be applied to situations. For example, visualize walking on nails. When the image of this painful situation is visualized clearly, you find yourself living and moving in a wholly different medium. The medium is dictated by pain in the feet. You find yourself walking gingerly, trying to apply even pressure on all parts of both feet so the nails

---

* Adapted from "Archetypes in Mime," *Mime and Beyond.* 40-1.

won't hurt any one part too much. The rest of the body reveals the pain. You must carry the image while you express it. Don't *act* it, but allow it to act on you.

Discover different media by visualizing walking through cold running water, over hot coals, through honey, and through glue that sticks to anything it touches. Visualize wet soap. No matter what part of the body touches the soap, it slips. Imagine a wall, a door marked "unknown," a tiger about to eat you. Swim into each image. Imagine being ten times taller than you are! Spend time with each new medium. Explore it and play with it. The freshness of an image is important. Don't interfere with the natural way the body is going to do it.

One must bring the image from that sphere of "no form" to "form." Once the body is trained to react and the image is visualized clearly, the body will reflect it faithfully. You must see the picture, be the picture, and allow the picture to be seen. In each case ask the question, "Do I *have* the image or *am* I the image?" Think movement!

When you use this technique to create a mime piece, the result is fantastic. There are six steps to doing a piece, and both archetypes and visualization can be used in each. First, know the material. This means know everything about the characters: why they are doing what they are doing, what sex they are, how old, where they live. Second, find the "how." Find the overall pattern, placement, and position of the pieces and internalize rhythms for the characters. Third, work the meaning, developing all the different levels inherent in the material. Fourth, develop the relationships between the characters and the sequences. Fifth, find the dramatic elements and the dramatic movements that will express them. Lastly, after all this is known, forget it and rehearse, rehearse, rehearse. When the piece is finally performed, do it as though it were being done for the first time.

A mime piece can be boring, interesting, or dramatic. If you know what you are doing, you don't waste any movement. If you are not yourself, the audience can't see itself. The audience can look at you, but it can't focus on you. Then, it gets bored. It becomes restless. If it is interested, it will remain calm. You must be a focus for the audience.

There must be continuity in thought and action. When you know the steps intuitively, then improvisation happens, not before. In that sphere of performance, you will burn to ashes if you are not pure.

When the totality of expression is understood, the mime performance becomes a focal point, a reflection that is active and centered. It communicates the multi-dimensional aspects of the self, soaring from abstract to concrete, from invisible to visible. That which is labeled by our three-dimensional limitations as "unknown" now becomes known.

GEOMETRICAL ECSTASY*

The perfect square has no corners. — Lao Tze

The mime is the geometrical human being in darkness. Without using her eyes she must know his line of movement and stay true to that line. She must also know the alignment of her body and its parts. She must see the form she wishes to create from within and project it with her body clearly. Only then can an audience experience her thought.

A mime does what mathematicians have been trying to do for all time: she actually squares the circle and circles the square. The rational is represented by the square. The circle represents intuition and feeling. To square the circle means to be rational, but with feeling. The body can do this both physically and non-physically. In mime, intellect marries intuition. The marriage or integration must be totally harmonious if it is to bear fruit.

We have a tendency to go to extremes. To circle the square we must have moderation. When a bell swings to its extremes, we hear a loud "bong, bong, bong." Only when it makes a tiny little swing in the middle do you hear a beautiful, subtle sound. This is the delicacy a mime achieves physically.

Like Euclidean geometry, the geometry of being has two axes, the horizontal and the vertical. Most of us take the verticality of our bodies for granted. We take for granted the steady horizontality of the floor where our feet are planted. We must take the most taken-for-granted things in life and study them. Mime allows us to see the axes and lines of our bodies.

Sometimes we use sticks to study line. A stick is like a fence. It gives you a geometrical line to move around. Although we do many exercises with the stick, we don't actually use it. We use the body. In a mime piece, a stick becomes an object outside ourselves. It can be a sword, an umbrella, a shovel, a door, a staff, a toothbrush, a fence. It can be anything. We can work, fight, love, and play with the stick. The task is to make the stick invisible, to make it disappear. By seeing the physical line of the stick we can see the non-physical line of our being, our double. It is the movement that happens around the stick that should be *seen*.

Any movement we do with one part of the body can be paralleled with a simultaneous opposite motion in another part. In pulling ropes, for example, the hands make one distinct geometrical line as they pull the rope across the body, and the pelvis moves in the opposite direction making a second line parallel to the first. The second line shows the motion of the body in relation to the rope. The movement is not just lines, but also the friction of those lines in opposition. Balance is the two opposites at work, pulling and pushing.

There are parallels all over the body: two legs, two arms, ribs, two lips, shoulders, nostrils, feet, toes, eyes. We see parallels everywhere we look — railroad tracks, walls, ceilings, floors, relationships, trees in the forest, traffic on the highway. Without parallels, nothing would exist.

Every movement has a line, a breath and a center. The effect of your breath flowing though the moving part of the body is like the effect of wind on a leaf. Our own center is like the center of a circle. It is the place where we know where we are. It is reality. It is the place we go out from and return to.

---

* Adapted from "Geometrical Mime," *Mime and Beyond.* 36-7.

When you know the center of a movement or where that movement originates, you can visualize the line that extends as the continuation of the movement. Thus, what appears to be linear reveals its natural non-linear quality. Wherever you stand, wherever you go is a center.

A mime artist has to be as sensitive as the antennae of a snail. When a snail senses sweetness it comes quickly with its slow, fluid motion. When it actually touches something it withdraws gently. The part that senses goes out and comes back into itself, as though taking back its breath. It has a rhythm that continues, echoing in space. The human body can learn to do this too, if it wants to. Lips that want to kiss will pull a head and neck toward another pair of lips. They anticipate the touch, kiss the space, and retract, withdrawing along the line of approach. Thus, by touching, one is touched. We don't have the patience or the resistance to stay in the transition. The snail can teach us to stay in the transit. If you learn the snail technique, you can write poetry with your body.

The snail doesn't work against nature, but with it. We don't imitate the snail, but we do try to learn from her ways. Here, our way of teaching mime is to return to nature. For example, a falling feather can teach you the way of the spiral. The spiral is the geometry of ecstasy. It is doing the circle step by step. All harmonious movements have a circularity about them. Nature is respectful to the circular. A circle reflects nature's cycles.

The body has its own laws, its own consciousness, and its own geometry. It is an architectural form — balanced and weighted. It is a structure very like a building, filled with tubes of all kinds that carry fluids, air, impulses and information. To be sure that the body's laws are experienced and learned, they have to be practiced. Observe, understand, and practice a law until it becomes yours. The intelligence that learns passes the information on to the one in you that knows. Geometrical ecstasy is conscious and controlled. It means being aware of lines, circles, avenues, and corridors of space. It means skilled delicacy. It means no random movement. That is geometry.

ON BEING ALERT *

Animals are instinctive: they have an ability to stay still, they have an immediacy of response, and they are naturally graceful and harmonious with nature. Animals know how to heal themselves. When wounded or sick, they withdraw and stop eating, licking the wound. Animals have many ways of communicating with one another. Their senses are sharp. Their movements speak. An animal stays alert because its degree of awareness determines its survival. The alternative to alertness is death.

Human beings have similar capacities, but don't choose to use most of them. A person's instinct speaks first in any situation, but the pushy intellect often gets in the way. It talks us out of following our intuitions. We rarely sit still as animals do or respond to situations immediately. Our bodies are naturally graceful, but we lose touch with them. When something hurts, we complain loudly and run to the doctor. We talk incessantly to one another, rarely listen, and thereby effectively block other natural means of communication. Our senses are dulled by lack of use. Although human beings have consciousness of their own mortality and animals seemingly do not, humans rarely behave with the moment-to-moment alertness that this knowledge demands.

The intellect loves to dominate. Its domination clouds the expression of our natural abilities. If you learn to turn the intellect off, when necessary, the abilities reassert themselves one by one. When you follow your true instinct, your actions usually succeed. Each of us has experienced the sharpening of our senses when we sit very quietly and focus our attention. Sounds we usually never notice emerge — birds, crickets, wind, water. They fill the space. The scents of moss, rich soil, or the hair of a friend suddenly become noticeable. We can feel thoughts and emotions from other people as clearly as if they were visible, tangible objects. And, little by little, many people are reawakening to their innate ability to heal themselves and to their ability to communicate in ways other than speaking.

It is the same with movement. When you *think* about doing a movement your mind is not still, and the body doesn't do the movement correctly. Instead, both the mind and the uninvolved area of the body need to stay still, but alert. The movement can then take place while "you" remain in the center of silence. This is the difference between thinking alert and being alert.

Being alert and moving without thinking are two important animal characteristics to study if we wish to understand clearly the "animal in us" and integrate that naturalness of movement into our own motions. Every animal has its own essence, every person has his or her own essence, every species has its genius. We can learn to run, jump, leap, and be still with animal genius. Apparently, to keep us humble, the only thing we can't do is fly.

When we study animals, many of our closed-minded attitudes and mental blocks, such as fear, insecurity, and game-playing are revealed. You can't fool an animal. It senses your fear immediately and reacts by taking a stance and preparing to attack. A mother bear freezes dead still when she first spots you. Do you respond without panic? Then perhaps she takes her cub and withdraws silently into the woods. You can approach any animal if you control your thoughts to that degree of purity where you see the sameness between yourself and the animal. Love the animal, and you will find that place of oneness between you. The animal becomes your teacher in that moment. You learn its essence and the language of its movement, and you see its characteristics in yourself.

---

* Revised from "On Being Alert," *Mime and Beyond*. 33-4.

To experience our animal characteristics and to sharpen our awareness, we do many exercises in our workshops at Le Centre du Silence. In "The Cat," catness pervades your being. "The Phoenix," condenses the lifespan of this remarkable bird into a few minutes. When the moment of its death approaches, the phoenix gathers palm fronds, arranges them around itself, and burns up in them. Out of the ashes arises a little phoenix. In this exercise you become a bird — you fly! You transcend the barrier of gravity between birds and humans, and you experience the legend on a physical level.

Other exercises develop individual senses like smell, sound, and touch. Can you recognize your friend with your eyes closed, using only your sense of smell? Does every centimeter of your skin touch and respond to touch with the same sensitivity your fingers have? When the senses awaken, refinement of the senses becomes possible. The result? Alertness, flexibility, balance, grace, and a host of other subtle faculties come into play. The body strengthens; every muscle and blood vessel responds. In the center of silence, movement speaks.

In yet another exercise, each student chooses an animal he or she is sympathetic with such as a cat, bird, elephant, or raccoon. The characteristics of that animal are transposed into the body. The student *becomes* that animal, following its behavior in its own setting. If you choose to be a bird, you hunt for worms, build a nest, sing to protect your territory, and fly. We don't imitate the animal, but we find the sympathetic meeting point between animals and humans and explore it.

Using the body as the medium for learning what the animal has to teach us, the exercises help students find inner resources that suggest their own inherent abilities to express themselves. When you allow yourself to "become" an animal, your body acts on a visceral level your intellect would otherwise never allow you to "stoop" to. Your natural behavior on this level reveals a whole, new, unexplored world that expands your repertoire of natural expression. It is a delightful and totally absorbing exploration of the self.

We learn to transpose animal characteristics into human ones. Performing a slothful person and performing a sloth in a forest are two very different things. Performing inadequacy and being inadequate are not the same thing either. You have to be articulate enough to show inadequacy adequately or slothfulness keenly. With this skill, students are able to deepen the meaning of each movement they make, because they bring it out of a primordial place within themselves. And then, the movement speaks.

BEING IN SPACE*

How do you fill a space? In writing on a piece of paper, you reveal yourself, not just by what you write, but by how you fill the space. Some people write from edge to edge. Others write only in the center. You are how you fill the space.

When a master makes a table, no nails or scraps of wood are left after he is finished. Everything is used. Everything is clean. Do not go to sleep at night until all the mistakes of the day have been corrected and the space is cleared. When some-thing is left undone or uncorrected, it creates tension. That tension keeps us uneasy until it is fully dealt with. The good carpenter straightens the bent nails.

Space is not a void. It is filled with thoughts, intentions and feelings. We always sense these, even if we don't acknowledge them. The ones not in accord with nature create tension. Wherever it is, tension attracts a kick.

A movement artist must be all eyes. We must learn to see with every pore like the blind. We *look* with the eyes; we *see* with the whole body. All the cells in the body have a consciousness and a specific function. There must be eyes in your toes, thighs, and belly. Walk as carefully forwards into the space as you do backwards. Don't walk, but be walked. There is a whole other world present to be experienced. Space awareness is an attunement that must be developed.

When we are in space we are like birds; we establish territories. How can you let the other person be in the space with you? Two people walking toward each other on a street often bump or disrupt their walking when they pass. There is no necessity for this if they simply give space to one another. When you walk, are you aware of the ants and the plants you step on? Do you trip and stub you toes? The feet, too, can learn to see.

At Le Centre du Silence, we do many exercises that develop space awareness quickly. For example, with your eyes closed, you must run across a floor covered with people lying down... and you must do this without kicking anyone. Another technique called "immediate replacement" develops the ability to fill a space the instant it is vacated by your partner, and in such a way that the tail of the imaginary line you create in space moves as one with the head of that line. By timing the space and spacing the time, each space is magically filled just as it is emptied. A kind of subtle contagion enflames a group when it perfects this attunement.

We also use sticks to test our alertness and our ability to respond immediately. Sticks let you see the amount of mercury you have in your blood. We roll the sticks in our hands, work combat maneuvers, exchange sticks in mid-air, and jump or duck to avoid getting hit. The body learns confidence and dexterity. It learns how to put only the exact amount of energy needed into motion. One iota of hesitation, fear or uncertainty can make the stick fall. Voila! It smashes your toe. Take care. If you overcompensate on one movement, you won't be ready for the next.

The stick teaches you how *not* to anticipate. It helps you give up all your expectations. The body and mind must be alert, both awake and quiet. The stick helps teach us that the right time to begin any movement is when all unnecessary movement stops and stillness descends.

---

* Revised from "Being in Space," *Mime and Beyond.* 29-30.

In each of us there is a witness or "one who observes." This observer is there whether you are aware of it or not. You begin to be conscious of the observer when you stop your unnecessary movements, are still, and listen to silence. When you allow the observer to watch over you, everything will be all right. Even if you are not conscious of it, it is conscious of you. It is the one who catches the body when it trips. You are always being taken care of.

The Inner Director lives in every cell. It is your double. A technique "75/25" teaches us to keep the observer always present and occupying 25% of our total being. It stays detached, witnessing, guiding the body. The observer lets us serve an idea, but keeps us from indulging in it. It saves us from accidents and fanaticism. Why doesn't an actor get carried away in a stage fight and really kill another actor? The observer keeps him aware of the truth and the still center within.

Another technique, called "Master of the Situation," teaches a whole group to act as one. It requires the members of the group to be fully conscious of the "one who observes" within themselves. Befriend the observer, and miracles happen!

When you allow your observer to be your director, you start to inhabit a space in a way that is both natural and conscious to you. There is purpose to the way you shape it. You can express eternity in a gesture. When your observer is always present, you begin to store up archetypes. In your storehouse are images common to human beings throughout the ages that provide the basis for a powerfully expressive common language of movement.

Speaking and thinking in archetypes and symbols also brings your thoughts and expressions to a level that is beyond linear. It breaks the logic of linear thinking. You sit peacefully and watch the train of thoughts go by. Suddenly, you jump on something. You choose. You say, "Ah, that's it!" A coalescence occurs. It is an alchemy of the spirit.

You are the laboratory. You are the experiment. You are the alchemist, the artist/scientist. You have to distill the chemicals in order to make the elixir. The more you mix, unify, and distill, the better artist/scientist you are. Use inner awareness. Always speak from the one in you who sees. Find your internal rhythm.

To be a Master of the Here and Now, that is the art of mime. The mime artist makes moments elastic; he squeezes time and elongates space. He studies the "elan" of a movement. He creates a space for something to happen *before* it happens. His observer keeps the image or happening in mind, and his body reflects that image. He fills space according to his awareness, and he shapes space according to his sensitivity. When he is finished, his workshop is clean. Space has been filled with meaning.

THE HARMONIOUS CELL*

The human body is a community of cells. It is a macrocosm made up of millions of functioning bits of matter. Each part has its unique work to do. Each cell has its own consciousness. Ears, liver, uterus, blood, vertebrae, muscle, tongue, tooth, heart; each part is vital to the totality.

In the same way, the cosmos is a community of cells made up of many elements. Each person is a dot in relation to the universe, but each dot has its unique place in the whole. A group of people is also a collection of cells.

No matter whether the being is single or many, it must be harmonious. In order to be one being, there must be a unifying thought or motif holding the pieces together. When a being or group is harmonious, it has a certain balance that is clearly visible. In order for this balance to manifest, each cell must know its place and its work. Each part must know *how* it is vital to the totality.

To express the totality, we must first perceive it. We have to overcome our usual elephant-in-the-dark-mentality. Six men in a dark room each got hold of a different part of one elephant, explored it thoroughly by touch, and then got together to discuss their six perceptions of "elephant." One described the trunk, another the ear, and another the tail. The other three told their perceptions of the leg, the back, and the tusk. Each was sure he knew what an elephant was, but no one could see the total picture. If the being is fully awake and lucid, each cell will move and act very consciously and will be aware of the totality. An ensemble must serve an idea in harmony. Each person must know his or her place within the ensemble. Everyone occupies territory. You choose your place to sit, and then you must accept your position because you chose to sit there.

When there is harmony in a person or group, thought is transformed into an image or form. A "physical mandala" is an example of such a transformation. Three or four people freeze into a harmonious form like a mandala. Then, at the exact same moment, the all begin moving very slowly, changing the structure. Suddenly, the motion simply stops — and miraculously, a new mandala is revealed. This can only happen when each member of the groups sees the whole picture. Each member must see not only his own perception, but everyone else's as well.

Every group contains leaders and followers, but the leader takes a certain initiative. An engine, for example, is the leader of a train. In movement, the initiating pulse or mark, is the leader. All the rest of the body parts are pulled along behind it like train cars following the engine. If the nose is the leader, it goes as far as it can on its own. Then, the head is pulled along after it. The neck follows, then the chest, waist and pelvis.

Walking uses two equal and perfectly blended leaders. Neither foot takes the lead. The leader was once where the follower is, and the follower will soon be where the leader is. It is simple. Accept that that which leads, leads and that which follows, follows. Any part of the body can be a leader. Any person in a group can be a leader. Just be careful not to allow the leader to become a dictator and the followers to become sheep.

Necessity is the leader of walking. An itch is the leader of scratching. Are you leading the movement, or is the movement leading you? A true leader is not seen. It does not make itself known. It

---

* Revised from "The Harmonious Cell," *Mime and Beyond.* 31-2.

remains hidden. As the root is hidden, the tree grows. When the blood stays in the body never to be seen, the body grows. In the same way, any leader should remain hidden. An audience doesn't want to see where the impulse to move in the group originates. And yet, in order to be hidden, you have to be very visible to those parts that must follow. It is because we stay tuned to that hidden leader that we succeed.

Mime is the only art form in which you can make the picture come out of the frame. You can make the sculpture breathe! The picture moves! The idea, the unifying thought, must be projected through movements. Every movement done by every person and every cell is **seen** by the audience.

A movement is a transition. In everyday life, transitions like taking the cap off the toothpaste happen too fast for us to see what takes place. In mime, movements are done slowly, one at a time, so they can be seen. Every movement must be done consciously in order for the idea to form. Every member of the group must know what part of his body or which person is the leader at any given moment. Each must give up some of his individuality to find the group balance. I can be her leg and she can be my arm! By moving consciously and by perceiving the totality, the invisible can be made visible.

If the ensemble is truly serving the idea in harmony, it should be as though one person were performing. Nothing happens until the right people with the right skills come together at the right time in the right place. Until all these things come together, we spend our time perfecting our skills and learning to listen. Then, when the right time comes, we'll be able to hear.

BEYOND OPPOSITES: *

The Electrical Journey Between Simplicity and Complexity

For everything that exists, its opposite also exists. We call this the Law of Polarity, I call it the "Bouncing Principle". All opposites exist simultaneously. Polarity means having both positive and negative. Without hard, no soft, without tension, no relaxation, without motion, no stillness. After inhaling comes exhaling, after contraction, expansion. The journey of this existence through simplicity and complexity, a sort of ball bouncing "up" and "down", between the "ceiling" and the "floor", and like an electrical spark in perpetual motion, we try to find balance and exist in a way, to find equilibrium between the two worlds, the "here" and "there", the "visible" and the "invisible". That's probably how the universe was born, through electrical impulses, a kind of conversation between matrices.

We really cannot perceive things unless we separate them. We divide and we divide, and the more we divide, the more we have the positive and the negative. We are here and we want to be there. Eventually the time comes when the dividing process stops. Division precedes uniting. There is a Oneness, one consciousness, underlying all things. One root. One beginning. Different manifestations, one essence.

Each of us has his own center which is like the center of a circle. It is the place where we know who we are. It is the place we go our from and return to, identical with the Center of all things, the One. Artists and mystics want to go directly to that center of things. When you work from there, you are solid as a rock.

An important part of our work is learning to be harmonious with opposites, or becoming, as we say, "lovers of paradox." This is indeed difficult, but unless we do it, we cannot enter the palace of true art. We are all limited beings, but we have to reach for the unlimited. Effort requires effortlessness. At the edge of ugliness is beauty.

In our mime work we learn to embody the paradox in thought and action. For example, we have to express weakness with strength. Our point of reference, the body, is a structure made of both the hard and the soft. It has the appearance of permanence; actually, it will die. This is a paradox we can play on easily. If someone hurts you, play the opposite: say thank you. Break the logic of life, and laughter or crying result spontaneously. That is when education happens. If a bullet hits you, don't die; pull it out, throw it back at the gunslinger, and watch it hit him! Accept the paradox, perform it, and then you transcend it.

In theater, there is the performer, the performed, and the performance. In thinking, there is the thinker, the thought, and the expression of the thought. These three are one. When we realize this, then we know totality. The paradox here is that the expression of totality happens through separation.

That which appears still, is essentially in motion, and that which appears to be moving is, in essence, still. The earth turns and the sun seems to move across the sky every day, but we don't notice its motion. We only see it now, above that tree, and then later, above that mountain. Each time it appears still. We

---

* Revised from "Beyond Opposites," *Mime and Beyond.* 38-9.

can't tell where the motion originates. A whirling dervish turns in a continual spiral, never wavering for an instant, but there is a profound stillness at his center that keeps him on one spot.

There are many other examples of this paradox in everyday life: the hub of a wheel turning, the eye of a hurricane, the frames of a film. When a person sits perfectly still, the blood continues to course through her body and breath fills and empties her lungs. Time is the fluid in which all this motion takes place.

There is no stillness on this earth. But in art, in painting, and sculpture, time is arrested. Moments are captured in space. These moments are the spaces *in between*. It is the work of the mime artist to perceive them. He is the sculptor of space, the shaper of force. His medium is space and time, and his paradox is that he must work simultaneously in the moment and in the timeless. The mime artist knows that he shares the same space and the same consciousness with all other beings. His work shows the marriage of subject and object. In order to know the architect, you have to know the architecture. The true mime artist must know the illusion of separateness so intimately that he ceases to be separate. When he sees the One, he is free to reflect all the forms of the duality of the world.

FACING THE MASK *

When a person covers his face with a mask, he thinks his real face is hidden. He feels safe behind the facade, and he acts as though he were not seen. Faces customarily dominate expression. We are accustomed to watching faces; consequently, we rarely notice what emotions the rest of the body is expressing. There are muscles in the face that we tense even when we think we are relaxed. When the gesticulations of the face are concealed by some sort of covering, a mask, suddenly we take notice of the body. Then something startling is revealed. By covering the face, we discover the real face, the real self.

Any appearance is a mask. Everyone knows that things are often not what they appear to be. Clothes, cars, jobs, routines, attitudes, and false smiles all mask the real person. Even personal history cloaks the real self.

Masks are the border between appearance and essence. At Le Centre du Silence we use plaster gauze to make white, neutral masks of our own faces. Neutrality is the space between yes and no. We use the masks to put the personality aside so we can find the *observateur* inside.

ON MAKING THE PLASTER MASK

Mask making is an insightful and deeply meaningful experience. The thoughts you carry while applying the wet gauze and shaping the face of your friend affect both his or her experience and your own intensely. Let calmness flow through your hands. Think good thoughts. Be gentle around the eyes and take care to leave two breathing holes at the nostrils. The life and death of your friend are in your hands.

As the mask forms on your face you encounter unique sensations. The large cheek muscles relax, the relaxed face relaxes the rest of the body, and the hardened mask feels strangely rigid against the relaxed face. You feel every centimeter of facial skin as you pull away from the hardened mask. Being in the hands of your friend in this special way allows real trust to be born between the two people.

When the mask comes off into your hands, you find yourself looking at the *inside* of your face. Your face lies in your hands before you, undeniably an outer limit, a mask. Behind that face lies the real you. The mask frees us to experience that real self.

---

* Revised from 'Facing The Mask" *Mime and Beyond.* 42-3.

HOW TO MAKE A MASK: INSTRUCTIONS

Read these instructions carefully prior to the mask-masking demonstration so that you may ask questions for clarification if necessary. Then review the instructions with your partner as part of your preparation for the mask-making. If you follow the instructions carefully, your mask will be a work of art and your experience of mask-making will be memorable.

Your purpose is to create a NEUTRAL life mask — neither laughing nor frowning — that captures an impression of your face in a calm, relaxed state. Though conforming to your face, the mask should have an archetypal appearance.

MATERIALS NEEDED
Vaseline, Water base Gesso
Fast-setting plaster bandage
Spackling paste
Acrylic paint (artist's quality in tube)
Matte-finish acrylic sealer (if desired)
A piece of narrow elastic

EQUIPMENT NEEDED
Fine-grade sand paper
Small stapler
A fine-hair broad water color brush
or foam "brush"
Scissors, Palette knife
X-acto knife (or similar tool)
Bowl, small finger nail file
Towel, paper tower, foam
Head and hair covering

Before beginning, allow a time of silence in which the person on whom the mask is being made can lie down and relax completely, allowing the facial muscles, in particular, to relax totally.

Avoid talking, outside noise, strong light during the making of the mask.

INSTRUCTIONS

1. Prepare, ahead of time, a bowl of lukewarm water and cut piece of plaster bandage into squares, triangles, thin strips, etc. (Large pieces for larger areas of face; small pieces for small areas of face.)

2. Spread Vaseline LIBERALLY over entire face.

    Pay particular attention to the eye areas and beard or moustache. Keep hair off face and covered.

3. Wet 1 piece of plaster at a time and stroke once or twice in a downward motion to dissolve the plaster smoothly and remove excess water. Gently tell the person where you are placing each

piece of plaster. Touch the face delicately, gently, mindfully, and with an attitude of complete respect.

4.   Systematically apply plaster pieces over the entire face.
PLACE THE PLASTER PIECES SO THAT THEY JUST TOUCH.
BE CERTAIN THAT THERE ARE NO OVERLAPS (overlaps create bumps). Do not push on the eyes.
Apply a second layer over the first (first layer need not be dry), being certain that the meeting places of the first layer are covered by the second layer.
DO NOT COVER NOSTRIL HOLES COMPLETELY. Drinking straws can be used in the nostrils as an aid if needed.
The mask will take 15-20 minutes to dry. Leave person lying quietly. **DO NOT** disturb him/her, as this may alter the facial expression.

5.   To remove the mask, sit up, put face in hands, and breath out of mouth slowly and gently into the mask until it falls into your hands.

6.   Allow the mask to sit over-night until dry.

7.   Cut around the edges to the form of your face, then, apply plaster strips around the mask edges to give a smooth appearance, and inside the eye edges.

8.   Cut out the eyes in the shape of almonds. Cut holes in the nostrils to breathe. **DO NOT TOUCH LIPS.**

9.   Sand well the mask lightly to get rid of roughness.

10.   Add enough water to spackling paste to form the consistency of thick cake batter. Spread a thin layer of spackling over the mask with the brush (or finger tips). You will need to apply 2 or 3 coats. Sand each layer. Although there is no need to wait until each layer is completely dry, it is best to let the spackling dry enough so that is doesn't stick to the sandpaper. Allow the spackling to dry completely before applying acrylic paint.

11.   Sand well before applying paint. Apply as many coats as you wish, using a fine-haired water-color brush or a foam brush. Use fingertips dipped in water to lightly smooth surface lines if necessary.

12.   Cut a piece of elastic band long enough to go around the back of your head, with approximately 1 and half inches left on each side for securing to the inside edge of the mask. Lay a strip of plaster over 1 inch of the elastic, leaving 1/2 inch free. Fold over this 1/2 inch to form a "V" that points into the face of the mask. Place another strip of plaster over this fold to secure it. Repeat on the other side of the mask.

ALWAYS USE THIN STRIPS OF PLASTER INSIDE MASK. DO NOT USE STAPLES OR PUNCH HOLES.

13.   For additional comfort, you may apply small pieces of foam inside mask. You may also apply spackling and acrylic sealer inside the mask for added strength.

14.   Write your name and the date inside the mask, it is a historic and a celebration moment in your life.

15.   May the experience of making your mask, and the mask session itself reveal for you the many facets of your unmasked being.

MASK SESSION
A Verbatim Transcript of the Mask Session

"Sit with the spine straight, in stillness. Hold the mask in your hands and look at it. Observe the texture and other details. It's part of your skin that you have peeled. It's a replica of your physical face. Think no thoughts other than about the mask. Look at the shape of the features. Do not judge, just look. Look at the eyes. They appear as two holes that reach infinity. Become familiar with your face that you hold in your hands.

"This tool, the mask, is a place. It's not a time. Become friends with the mask and it will teach you many things. Your face is looking at you. It is covered, somehow, by different thoughts.

"Very slowly put the mask on your face. Take five million years to do this. No brusque movements. Every movement should be very conscious. With the mask on, keep the eyes closed. Breathe very calmly. Begin to feel your own facial structure under the mask. It is covered, as if by clothes.

"Visualize yourself sitting in water up to your neck. It is the ocean. What you see is the horizon of the waters. Nourish the waters, the horizon, and ask who is behind the mask. It has no name. Is it your face? Is the mask really that important, or is it just a tool to help us realize the essence? No attributes, no name, no concept — totally pure. If we can grasp that ungraspable, then later we can express that essence.

"Find the neutral one, the no-name one, the circle, the empty one within. That center of the circle is there living behind every being.

"Open the eyes halfway. What you see on the other side of the horizon is the reflection of yourself. Be detached from it. There is no such thing as near or far. You cannot measure the horizon. The water is cool and helps the body in that total peace.

"In very slow motion, like moving for the first time, check to see if the mask is still there. The hands don't touch as if they know, they touch as if they want to know. Look at your hands through the windows of your eyes.

"Stand up using very slow motion. Who is behind the mask moving the body? It is a new physical being that you discover, but who is discovering it? Who is moving the body from the inside? The goal is to stand. Do not plan any movement. Let the one behind the mask move you.

"Once you stand, get in touch with that presence. The presence is not you. It's no-name. If we are aware of it, everything becomes fresh, as if for the first time. Let the presence walk, using the vehicle of the body. Any movement we do now is in the service of walking, with appreciation and reverence. The presence goes for a promenade. It is not limited in any way. Turn. When the head meets the limitation of the body, the presence continues. The presence will teach you to turn.

"Now we take certain conditions and see how the presence relates. Be cold! Let coldness contract the body, as the presence stays remote, observing the expression of the body. Watch how the mask keeps the face from interfering in the body's expression. Now change; be hot! Immediately the body expands and droops, but the presence stays distant.

"The body takes on archetypes. Be a warrior! The archetype of the warrior is one who knows his power and knows how to use it positively. Be a coward! Receive the universal coward in you. Cowardice is not negative; it is a state of being. Let the presence teach you how to use the body as a brush. Presence never needs to justify itself. The presence knows.

"Come back to the original spot where you began. The presence sits like a king or queen. It knows how to sit. The one who is sitting has a right to be there. Turn the head to brush the horizon. Just the head. C'est une noblesse de presence. Close the windows and sit still in the waters. Very slowly, eyes closed, take off the mask and hold it facing you."

The work with masks opens beautiful doors to us to be in touch with ourselves and to become aware of the presence, that formless guidance, that springs up from the center of our being. This form of work opens new vistas of self exploration to the student. Further, it provides specific tools to enter into the inner self, learn, experience, and emerge with a definitive artistic expression.

THREE PILLARS
OF BECOMING AN ARTIST*

A Journey from Thought to Action

INTRODUCTION

It is not innate in the human character to dwell deeply in the heart of any subject by inquiring into it, research and truly mastering all facets of the subject. Especially now, in our time, when this society willingly accepts mediocrity and the appearance, rather than the actuality of excellence. People are not generally encouraged to develop more than one per cent of their learning potential of a subject or an art.

Therefore, it is advisable for the serious future artist to ask the right questions and to have the model of his goal very clearly in mind, for he or she will receive little reinforcement from the surroundings. He or she must be prepared for dedicated study. It is only in the repetition of the craft that he or she masters the art. Only when the craft becomes second nature can one begin to create from his or her inner being the forms, images and conceptions to create within that art.

In mime, as in other arts, the student must discover himself. He needs to recognize how the Law of the Triangle applies to his study, as to any art. Just as the seed first roots, grows tall and flowers, and finally bears fruit, so does a student learn, discover, and finally create within his or her art.

The student passes through three stages, three points of the triangle; the *"Three Pillars of Becoming an Artist."* At the first point of the triangle of an *apprentice;* the **SKILL** is mastered. At the second point of the triangle, the student is a *craftsman.* He applies what he has learned to the **CRAFT**. These two initial developmental stages culminate in the third point, wherein, the student, artist, or master, creates the **ART**.

The vision of these three pillars, **SKILL**, **CRAFT**, and **ART** could encourage the student to become an artist. A conscious functional being who transforms the world he perceives via his art, sharing his expertise and his inspiration in his presentation of an inner vision that transcends the finite.

SKILL

In order to become an apprentice, one must already want to learn and be willing to pursue his or her chosen art by undertaking the necessary tasks to master it. Few people are willing to dedicate themselves to the long and arduous path to the mastery of an art, and few are willing to place themselves in the apprenticeship of a teacher.

A human being is like a seed. Every human being is endowed with gifts from the mother and father. These gifts are the being's talents. These talents are his or her sustenance and nutrition, just as the food for the potential plant is already contained in the seed. The wise farmer who nurtures the see is like the teacher.

When a person decides to become an apprentice to an art, he or she takes root. When a seed roots, it pushes away from the warming sun into the resisting earth, searching blindly, pushing all obstacles away. The apprentice does the same. The farmer provides the necessary nutrients and a steady flow of water. The teacher does the same. The root must receive the nutrients and must learn to differentiate between what is good and bad for it. It must struggle within the earth's confines.

The teacher gives various tasks to the qualified apprentice. The student must master the techniques of the art. He or she must become a physical technician, learning to "play the instrument." For the mime student, the instrument is the physical body. Balance, gesture, and clarity of expression must be mastered. The student learns specific skills through trial and error. He learns one thing at a time. He sharpens his tools. He deals with the ego, taking direction from others in the correct manner of doing.

The apprentice must trust and depend upon the eyes of the teacher. The teacher provides circumstances that reveal the random tendencies and incomplete efforts of the student. He also provides circumstances for the student to experience artistic inspiration. Artistic inspiration is like the sun. It warms the apprentice/root and urges it onward. It inspires the apprentice to aim his sights high, usually beyond his capacity to realize.

Thus, apprenticeship is a dark and difficult period. The student does not see where he is going. Being still "underground," the student makes many mistakes, often resulting in shame, fear, self-blame and hostility to the work. In the desire to advancement of skills, urgency and impatience tend to make the student seek short cuts, which limit the full development of the skills.

This resistance is very important for the continuation of life. It saves the student from harm, but it also holds him back from accomplishing what he can. Students can be resistant to different things including the task, the teacher, and other students, trying, and succeeding, failing, testing, exertion. If the student does not do the tasks set for him; he will not learn the lesson. Teachers need a great deal of patience, for it often takes students a long time to overcome their resistance.

The apprentice struggles with self-discipline, with learning what nutrients to absorb, and with his or her habits. As with the root, this is done in darkness, without knowledge of the end and without reward. The tasks provided by the teacher are suited to individual growth. For example, in mime, the student must continue to do physical exercise daily. He must learn the involuntary processes of the body. He must train the body and the imagination with a variety of both repetitive and new tasks. One root is not enough. One skill is not sufficient for the apprentice. The more struggle, the more roots, the stronger the plant.

When the student is able to perform any tasks without resistance or negativity, then, he or she is able to develop the needed skills for self-expression. Only when the skills become second nature, will the apprentice be ready for the next stage in the development of the artist – **The Craft.**

CRAFT

When a person makes the transition from apprentice to craftsman, it is like the seedling that finally breaks through the earth into the sun and the air. The root has penetrated the earth deeply, conducting water and nutrients back to the seed in order finally to split it open.

The food within the seed is consumed, destroying it. But this very act begins the upward growth of the sprout. This vertical growth is the last effort of the apprentice. When the tiny plant breaks the earth, a great transition takes place. Before this event the plant knew only vertical growth, down and up. It knew only itself.

When it breaks into the air the seedling/ apprentice suddenly sees the world all around it. This view is staggering. It realizes that there is a horizontal as well as a vertical. It realizes that it is an insignificant little being in a large and indifferent world. It is real effort is just beginning.

The transition to craftsman begins when the student realizes this relationship he has to the world. His apprenticeship, which had been a source of resistance, is now seen as a solid base to build on. Thus, when a student becomes adept enough with his art, opportunities present themselves, which require him or her to make use of the skills. This can happen in many ways. The teacher may see that the student is ready and start to use him or her in ways demanding a synthesis of skills. The student might get a job requiring a similar synthesis. There exists a law of supply and demand in the universe such that when a need appears, simultaneously one appears to fill that need.

When a thing transmutes, such as in the changes from apprentice to craftsman, it changes its arena. The fledging craftsman takes the skills and puts them into some context. In the case of the mime craftsman, he or she begins to apply the physical and imaginative skills that have become second nature by creating productions. These are performed, tested by fire, before audiences. If the ideas work, the craftsman continues. If not, he or she reroutes the work.

The work of the craftsman is very visible. He is very much in the world. He is a master of technique and he learns to apply it to perfection. He works to perfect his art. The craftsman is an organizer; he is adept, but not necessarily inspired. He goes to seek his own horizon. He examines his own personal cycles and then learns the rules or cycles of the universe. If the conditions are favorable, the plant grows very tall and strong, putting out foliage and beautiful flowers. The downward growth of the roots continues. The roots continue to feed the adult plant. Many natural disasters may befall the plant as it continues to reach toward the sun.

The craftsman continues to be a student. He may begin to teach other students the basic skills. He can see from where he has come and to where he is going. He must withstand many tests: high wind, scorching heat, and bitter cold, lack of nutrition, lack of water. But the question for the plant always remains - will it bear fruit?

The craftsman labors day and night. He fashions his sustenance by day and receives the medium of expression by night. Only if he is conscious of this can he proceed toward becoming transformed. If this consciousness is not fully developed, he will become ordered, efficient and versatile, but not inspired. He will remain a perfect closed system, but will not allow the creative impulse to enter from the unknown.

ARTIST

The artist is the one who steps into the unknown and acts as though it was just another day. In order for the plant to perpetuate it self, it must bear fruit. The seeds must be scattered to the winds, falling invisibly in many places, then growing silently to foster new plants to bear new fruit. The development of the fruit is imperative to the continuation of the cycle.

The great challenge to the aspirant artist is the balancing of the physical and the inspiration. When the student/craftsman develops into the artist, he must become receptive to the unknown, the unseen. He must search for his source, the essence of his original seed. But the world, sophisticated and fast moving, never encourages such an inner search.

A plant does not bear fruit unless all the conditions and the growth are balanced. If the growth of foliage parallels the advance of root growth, there is promise. If the plant blooms too early, the subsequent loss of energy brings premature death. Threats to the organism can cause stasis, in the case of the craftsman becoming artist, rigidity and caution. If the leaves grow too luxuriantly, the plant grows abundantly beautiful, but it does not produce fruit. Such stalks have the appearance of fertility, but the lack of purpose in their efforts shows them to be merely vigorous.

The artist must provide continuity for the invisible. He or she is a pure vessel and is always alone. Inspiration comes from being cognizant of the natural order of the world. The artist seeks what is behind the veil, and in doing so, gets in touch with the creative light - the Sun. The artist is like anyone else, but in his deepest being, he is a creator knowing all the steps a student must take. The artist has experienced time as well, and has learned how to condense actions and thoughts very speedily. In doing so, the artist works beyond time. He is every-changing, yet precise. He can create and transform beyond all techniques. The techniques he has mastered are only aids to the self-expression he reaches for deep within himself. He creates the forms, images and conceptions that form the art from his inner being, reaching the highest in people. He acts unexpectedly, transcending skills, creating surprises, fusing life and art.

The student/artist knows HOW to learn; never forgetting that one ceases to be an artist when one stops learning. He must discover for himself the additional learning task he faces. Being an artist requires great self-discipline and sincere dedication.

The artist is challenged to invent new ways to symbolize and communicate ancient truths. He must stay in touch with his source through attunement to spiritual reality in order to discover the ultimate creativity in himself. He is a transformer. He has merged the personal and the impersonal into a transcendent level, a measure of both, in harmony and unison. In doing so, he works on many levels at once, touching everyone. He transforms raw material to gold.

The mime artist shapes the invisible space. He or she achieves unity between himself and all present in the audience by tuning the vibrations with his actions. To do this the artist must discover not only his own rhythmic inner music, but that of the whole audience as well. He is able to do this because mime, or any art, originates from the depths of silence, from the self-search for cosmic expression of the essence of life, which is in all. Thus, the artist opens new spaces in our consciousness by being a mirror of the epoch. The members of the audience see themselves and are transformed. Through the union of the mime artist-audience, mind-body, an individual-group consciousness is achieved.

CONCLUSION

We have seen how the Law of the Triangle applies to the Three Pillars of Becoming an Artist. The third point, the artist, is built on the synthesis of the other two: *The apprentice and the craftsman*. All students have various tasks facing them. The apprentice is given tasks by his teacher or situations, which he faces with a certain amount of resistance. The apprentice learns the skills necessary in order to know the self and others. The tasks of the craftsman appear before him in the application of the skills he has learned as an apprentice. He discovers and sets new tasks for himself, and contributes from his creative process to the world.

The artist must persevere beyond the limited conventions and the unexamined assumptions consciously and continuously. He draws inspiration from the inner creative source and works invisibly, planting new seeds in the world, presenting an inner vision that transcends the finite, and creates something new that was not there before.

* From *Mime and Beyond: The Silent Outcry by Samuel Avital* (Pages 6-10)

HANDS *
The Instrument of Creation

In mime and in dance, hands design the space and sculpt the air. From one creative impulse, the air is given movement, the space takes shape, by simple movements.

The Uniqueness of the Human Hand**

The hand exhibits one of the most important distinctions between human beings and other animals. It has profoundly influenced our evolution, enabling us to create works of art and feats of engineering.

The arboreal life of our ancestors encouraged the development of this efficient grasping mechanism, capable of performing delicate manipulations. The sense of touch sharpened and indirectly enabled our progenitors to judge distance and direction more accurately. When early hominids descended from trees, the prehensile hand, now free, became the main exploratory tool.

Primates, including humans, lost their claws early in their evolutionary ascent. But of the primates, only humans can join the tip of the index finger with an opposable thumb. Due to the maneuverability and dexterity of the thumb and fingers, humans gained a precision in grasping small objects and a lightness of touch, and thus a facility with the use of tools that would be impossible with claws.

We owe the architectural and functional excellence of the hand to an intricate system of muscles, a metacarpal (palm bone), and phalanges (finger bones). Around and within the layers of ligaments, fibers, and tissues that stabilize this skeletal structure, there is an intricate network of muscles that makes possible the amazingly versatile motor performance of the hand.

The prehensile action of the hand makes two basic movements possible: the precision grip and the power grip. The first permits accuracy and fine control. The second is a posture of labor, in which the entire hand holds an object between the flexed fingers and the palm while the thumb supplies the necessary pressure to maintain the grip.

A network of nerves of the fingers transmit heat or pain and convert the mechanical energy of touch into electric energy that is carried by the nerves to the higher centers. Other more sensitive neural tactile receptors permit discrimination among objects. Even the fingerprints with their unique configuration of whorls, loops, and arches, assist the fingers to grip and pick up objects.

The thumb and fingers are primary organs of the vast human sensory system. A relatively large area of the brain governs them. The thumb, for instance, is governed in the brain cortex by an area almost as large as that which controls the entire hip and leg.

---

* Adapted from "Hands — The Expression of the Soul," *Mime and Beyond*. 135-6, and from an unpublished manuscript.

** See also the discussion of "**So What** "in "Defintuitions" and "In Brief, Samuel's Small Words for Big Things."

The Awareness of Touch - Hands Exercises

Human beings have very highly developed eye-hand coordination, the hands responding instantly to silent messages from the brain, informed by the eye. But the very delicate pressure sensors (propioceptors) in our fingertips enable us to know when we are approaching an object, even without the assistance of our eyes. This is how, for example, we can close our eyes and touch the tip of our nose. Even the most sophisticated robot cannot begin to match this kinesthetic capability, which we take for granted. To become aware of the subtle capabilities of the hands we suggest a few exercises:

1. Rub the hands very vigorously for about a minute until you feel heat created by friction. Inhale and raise your hands over your head. Feel the generation of energy flowing through the body.

2. Once again, rub the hands very vigorously for a minute. Then place the palms in front of you as if you were holding a ball about six inches in diameter. Feel the lines of force, like the lines of force of a magnet, connecting the hands. Now slowly bring the hands together until they almost touch. Do you feel the tingling? Do any "sparks" leap the gap between your hands? Now s-l-o-w-l-y pull your hands apart until the lines of force snap, just as do the lines of force in a bar magnet when the poles are pulled apart and then suddenly release. How far apart are your hands when you feel the snap?

3. Clap the hands lightly for about a minute in such a way that the palms and all the fingers meet. Then, with the arms at a right angle, shake the hands at the wrists in a variety of motions — up-and-down, side-to-side, towards each other, away from each other — for several minutes. Finish by dropping the hands at your sides. Discover for yourself the intensity of the energy concentrated in them by the tingling sensation of sparks shooting out the ends of the fingertips.

4. Stand facing the sun in the morning and stretch the arms to shoulder level. Close the fists, contracting the fingers, and then open the fists, stretching the fingers. Do this for one minute and feel the result. After performing any of these hand energizers, touch an object s-l-o-w-l-y, as if for the first time. What new sensations do you discover?

5. Stand erect. Stretch the right arm forward until the hand is at shoulder level, then extend it straight out to the side at shoulder level, and then let it come back down to your side. Repeat this with the left arm. This exercise is especially good for coordination of the right-left crisscross of energy in the body.

6. Practice the Fish Wave, a wavy movement in which the hand is taught to undulate like a fish.

    Begin with the palms together, fingers touching.

    Second, fan the fingers, keeping the palms together.

    Third, cup both hands away from each other, keeping fingertips and heels of the palms touching.

    Fourth, bring the first knuckle joints together, leaving the outspread fingers still cupped.

    Fifth, slowly stretch the fingers up until the whole hand is flat against the other once again, and then allow the fingers to peel outward as far as possible from each other, like the petals of a flower opening.

Finally, bring the palms together as in the beginning and repeat the exercise many times. Eventually do it with one hand alone in space, moving it in many different directions — vertically, horizontally, diagonally, right-to-left, left-to-right — like a fish swimming.

With continued practice of this exercise, your hands will become remarkably supple and responsive. You will be able to touch with greater sensitivity and have a fuller appreciation for tactile nuances.

By increasing our awareness of the hands through exercises, we come to realize that they are actually transmitters of energy and of the knowledge in which our fluid thoughts take form. If we take this into consideration, we will see a positive transformation in our lives. Every moment and gesture becomes of utmost importance to us. We gain poise and calm envelops all life within and without. We will then write our poems on the walls of history with these hands.

It is said that when the hands are flexible, it is a sign of spiritual flexibility. An ancient Chinese exercise of pushing the fingers backwards makes them flexible so that the spirit will also be flexible. The ancient Greeks would test children's hands for flexibility to see if they had the potential to become artists.

The attainment of high spiritual powers by the individual has been associated with certain postures of the body, especially hand gestures, which not only aid concentration, but are capable of evoking the inner spiritual consciousness.

The Hindus have devised a highly formalized and cultivated gesture language, Kathakali, a grammatically complete language of hand symbols or mudras, regarded to be expressive of spiritual states and the qualities of deities. The palm, for example, symbolizes the calm center of action, the meditative control over the five senses or fingers agitated around it. One hand held up, palm outward, is known as "turning the wheel of the law." It is also a teaching position. The hands held together indicate the begging bowl.

Some of these gestures, apart from their spiritual significance and symbolism, are wonderfully articulate, with a grace and tenderness of poetic expression, and capable of depicting any theme, situation, emotion, or action required. Each theme has its own sequence of hand positions and movements, with coordinated attitude and body movements based on certain archetypal or idealized forms.

The opening lotus bud, for example, is shown, not only by a single symbolic gesture, but also by a series of hand movements, beginning with a cyclic twist of the hand to suggest the very growth of the flower, followed by delicate movements of the fingers to indicate unfolding petals. Visualize for a moment an Indian dancer, her hands fluttering to indicate water, the flight of the bee, or the opening of a lotus. An undulating hand suggests waves, or a fish; a swinging hand creates elephant ears or the flight of a bird; and a shaking hand shows anger, a river, rising flames, or lightning. These movements of the hands are thought to represent divine actions, being distinguished in their conventions from the movements and gestures of ordinary human beings.

Native Americans evolved elaborately codified ceremonial sign languages which yet retain a beautiful mimetic simplicity and directness. A ceremonial dancer, for example, shades his eyes to see into the distance. This action is repeated toward the four points of the compass as the dancer looks toward the approaching rain gods who bring the rain. He may also enact motions of sowing seeds, digging, and gathering plants. Native American animal dances are highly mimetic, imitating the flight of geese or eagles or the supernatural powers of bears or bison.

41

Many traditional ceremonial hand gestures also prevail in the Christian church. The thumb and first two fingers raised represent the Trinity and are used by the Pope in blessing the faithful. The arms outstretched form a cross with the body, expressing suffering in life and death.

The seated Buddha calls the earth to witness with a downward pointing right hand, while receiving from above with an upturned left hand laid in his lap. Similarly, dervishes whirl with the left palm extended upward to receive from heaven and the right palm facing the earth to transmit the energy through their bodies to the earth.

At ancient Egyptian funeral ceremonies, the hands held palms upward above the head signified the rising of the soul; holding the arms in a gesture of throwing dust on the head indicated mourning; arms held directly upward signified interceding with the gods for the dead; a pushing movement sent threatening evil spirits away from the dead.

In the Hebrew tradition the hand is the connector through which the spirit may touch matter, and with which we may touch spirit with matter while living in the flesh. In Hebrew, the word for hand is Yad. Yod, the first letter of Yad, is the tenth letter of the Hebrew alphabet and designates the ten fingers.

Now Yad numerically in Hebrew equals 14, designating the 14 phalanges of the human hand. We have two hands, equaling 28 phalanges. The number 28 creates the word Koah, meaning "power," the power that we possess in our hands or actions.

The hand is also our point of contact with others; we shake hands to make contact with a friend — two hands come together. In Hebrew, the word Yadid, meaning "friends," is spelled Yad Yad, which also adds up to 28, power. So the power of two hands is friendship. And in joining hands we gain a mighty power to create and expand.

THE FOUR LONGEVITY CYCLES

"The more I learn the more I realize I don't know,
and the more I realize I don't know, the more I want to learn."
Albert Einstein

The Body*Speak*™ workshops introduce a method of training developed to cultivate moment-to-moment attention to action. Working individually and in groups, we study the relation of motion and stillness, explore groundedness and gravity, break down movements into their finest components, and employ the ultimate object —a simple stick—to redefine our concepts of verticality and connection.

We also introduce the daily practice of four powerfully integrative and essential sets of exercises to enhance longevity and joie de vivre known as The Longevity Cycles.

THE LONGEVITY CYCLES

1. **Flexibility Cycle (1)**   Gently limbers and focuses the body
2. **Regenerative Cycle (2)**   Integrates physical, mental and emotional attention to lubricate and regenerate the entire organism.
3. **Integrative Cycle (3)**   Balances and focuses your life force and theatrical skills.
4. **Self-Evolutionary Cycle (4)**   Develop balanced self-guidance, and quickens your personal evolution.

The Longevity Cycles are offered through private sessions to individuals and special group workshop sessions. Programs are offered in Boulder, Colorado and around the world, or via phone or email.

THE FLEXIBILITY CYCLE (1)

The Flexibility Cycle (1)

Gently limbers, make flexible, and focuses all parts of the body; a journey through the spine and the skeleton to be familiar and at ease with movements that could help the body to live longer.

Cycles 1 through 4 are introduced live by Samuel during the **BodySpeak™** workshops. If you practice from these notes, make sure to follow the instructions carefully.

<u>**Key:**</u>   **R = right   L= Left   U = up   D = down   F = front   B = back**

1. **ZERO**   Standing vertically in balance, spine straight, eyes on horizon, hands down, shoulders back, chin in, feet parallel.

2. **HEAD**
   a. **EGYPTIAN PROFILE** , RL x 10, UD x 10
   b. Circle R x 3, L x 3

3. **EYE COMPASS**   RCLC/UCDC, Diagonal URC/DLC
   Diagonal ULC/DRC x 3, Circle R x3 , L x 3

4. **SHOULDERS**
   a. Shake UD x 10
   b. Right UD - Left UD x 10
   c. Both Right-Left U - Both Right-Left D
   d. Circle both shoulders x 5
      One after the other x 5

5. **ELBOWS**
   a. Hands fixed on wall, rotate elbows x 10
   b. Right Hand in left palm, full circled w/elbow x 10
   c. Left Hand in right palm, full circled w/elbow x 10

6. **WRISTS**
   a. Both wrists UD x 20 (toward center)
   b. Alternate, accelerate RL x 20 - UD x 20
   c. Lift arms and hold, hands down slow, exhale

7. **THE BEAUTIFUL CURVE**
   Lift arms curved (with elbow fixed with arms
   as one unit) in "willow" position overhead, hands mark open and outward position.
   Caress space (palms outward) as you bring your arms down sideways, maintaining the beautiful curve, gracefully.

8. **SUN MOON EXERCISE**
   Hold both hands palms facing each other
   together at chest position, lift R-U and L-D together and back L-U and R-D and back to chest, first position. repeat the cycle x 5

9. **CHEST**
   a. Inclination RL x 10, FB x 10
   b. Inclining circle R x 5, L x 5
   c. Translation RCLC x 10 FCBC x 10
   d. Translating circle R x 5, L x 5

44

| 10. **WAIST** | a. Deep inclination RL x 10 FB x 5 |
| | b. Deep circle R x 5, L x 5 |

11. **PELVIS**	a. Shoulders remain level, heel of working leg lifts, toes remain on floor. Lift hip R x 5, L x 5, RL x 5
	b. DOUBLE PINS, pelvic rotation FB x 10
	c. small circles, hands clasped behind head R x 5. L x 5
	d. Big circles, hands on back on the hip R x 5, L x 5

| 12. **TWIST** | Bend knees, feet shoulder width apart, hands clasped behind head R and L x 10 |

| 13. **KNEES** | Empty the knees, one after the other, as if collapsing slightly R and L x 10 |

| 14. **ANKLES** | a. Activate ankles while standing on opposite leg Right FB x 10, Rotation Left FB x 10 |
| | b. Make circling motions with ankles, each foot Rotation R x 10, Rotation L x 10 |

| 15. **RUNNING IN PLACE** | Begin walking quietly in place, accelerate gradually to running in place, lifting knees, then decelerate back to quiet walking until stillness. |

| 16. **KICKING** | Coordinate leg kick with thrust of opposite arm, R and L x 10. Right initiates FB and Left initiates FB x 10 |

| 17. **FIRE** | Gradual shaking from bottom of feet as if catching fire. The whole body shakes (with self control). Then stop sharp, exhale, rest. repeat x 3 |

| 18. **WHIRLING** | Turning around axis with movement directed from hip center, Swing arms several times like empty sleeves. Then whirl on axis R to L direction for a few turns. Return to center, Always initiate movement from the pelvic center. |

19. RELAXATION AND MENTAL REVIEW

Position your knees and feet together, lower to sitting position. Lower back of legs simultaneously to the floor.
Stretch body in relaxed supine position, palms up. Now calmly, still and silent, do a mental review of of the entire cycle, see yourself doing it as if you are watching yourself.

20. LIGHTNING

From the relaxation position, come to attention. First sit upright quickly, then stand, extend hands above head and inhale (like a zigzag of a lightning bolt).

Exhale, caress space. and do The Beautiful Curve.

THE REGENERATIVE CYCLE (2)

Regenerative Cycle (2) Integrates physical, mental and emotional attention to lubricate and regenerate the entire organism through simple yet powerful exercises that proved to be very effective in the last 30 years of practice by thousands of Le Centre Du Silence students worldwide.

Key: R = right   L= Left   U = up   D = down   F = front   B = back

1. **GREETING** Clapping hands, applauding one another and ourselves, taking a bow in circle formation

2. **INTEGRATION MOVEMENT** This movement seals each step of the cycle, linking t to the next.

   - From Earth — tap hands on ground
   - Though Me — clap hands together
   - To Heaven — stretch hands outward
   - Exhale, hands down with **the Beautiful Curve.**

3. **BODY TAPING** With rhythmic breathing: 2 taps — exhale.
   Tap arms, shoulders, chest, abdomen, legs, back, rub kidneys & intestines areas, rub hands and nails.

   DO THE INTEGRATING MOVEMENT

4. **APPLE STRETCH** Pick the apple; eat it; exercise jaws, teeth; throw the seed back to earth at the center of the circle.

   DO THE INTEGRATING MOVEMENT

5. **ARMATURE**
   a. Elbows bent at shoulder level; bring back and meet shoulder blades twice with 2 inhales.
   b. Arms at 45 degree angle down; back twice with 2 inhales.
   c. Windmill arms R x 10, L x 10, both x 10, alternating x 10.
   d. Arms swings — eyes soft focus to horizon; knees slightly bent; feet parallel; 2 inhales, 2 exhales x 100+

6. **HOLDING THE EARTH** Arms rounded, holding the ball of the earth; swing toward ground RL x 4, then up to R, repeat sequence to L, R, L, bow to each other in greeting gestures. Improvise, be creative.

7. **RAG DOLL** Bend over forward, hand & head loose like a doll release, shake out with exhaling sound.

8. **SILLILAND** Squat to do face massage, tapping as follows:

a. Around the eyes, temples, cheeks, nose, nostrils points, lips, tongue; growl and stretch the face with fingers;

b. **"Moroccan goat propeller"**. Hold chin with left hand, hold the left small finger with your right thumb, and shake hands, chin, like a propeller, make sound, release breath.

c. Massage the ears, cup hands over ears, listen to the inner sounds, hum, be quiet, absorb, focus on breathing.

9. **SOLE DRUM**

a. Sit with legs together and straight; hold toes and stretch RL x 10, legs apart RL x 10

b. Cross ankle over opposite knee, vigorously tap the sole of the foot, massage around ankles; repeat same with the other leg.

10. **BICYCLE, SCISSORS AND CIRCLE**

Recline on elbows or flat on back, hands under buttocks for support.

a. bicycle RL x 20

b. scissors RL x 20

c. leg circles (inward) x 20, (outward) x 20

11. **ROCK THE BABY**

Cradle right leg with both arms; left leg out-stretched, twist, rock sideways RL while singing the French song **"A la Claire Fontaine"** repeat same for left leg.

12. **LION'S ROAR**

Sit with one leg over the other (half lotus), cross arms, grasp opposite knee, inhale, stretch up, exhale, growling down like a lion claiming the kingdom. Release all body tensions.

13. **CAT STRETCH**

From squat position: extend legs, keeping hands on floor. Walk forward with hands to inverted "V" position. Stretch legs by alternating lifting heels RL x 10. Walk forward with feet. Hold toes. Stretch up from pelvis slowly. Stand up. Repeat x 5.

14. **SALUTATION TO YOURSELF**

Stand erect, rub ankles together while massaging the breast points (several times). Then say silently with accompanying movements:

- I reach my hands to the world.
- I open myself to new experiences.
- I take a step toward life.
- I expend myself with the universe.
- I give more than I receive.
- I come back to myself enriched and integrated.

NOTE:

Movements, postures, attitudes and instructions for #14 are demonstrated during the workshop.

Until you learn them in person at the **Body*Speak*™** workshops, improvise on your own, be creative, integrating the word with the movement according to your understanding.

THE INTEGRATIVE CYCLE (3)

Integrative Cycle (3)   A profound sequence of subtle movements to balance and focus your life force and theatrical and communicative skills.

This cycle contains in essence a condensed version of all the **Body*Speak*™** techniques, philosophies, postures, attitudes, mental and physical integration.

<u>**Key:**</u>   **R = right   L= Left   U = up   D = down   F = front   B = back**

1. **HEAD AND EYES**

a. **EYE COMPASS (Eye movements)**
RCLC - UCDC - Diagonal URC - DLC
Diagonal ULC - DRC X 3
Circle R X 3 - Circle L X 3

b. **LEADERS/FOLLOWERS (Eye movements)**
Eyes leads, head follows
RC - LC, UC - DC X 3
Head leads, eyes follows
RC - LC, UC - DC X 3

c. **SOFT EYE - SHARP FOCUS**
Eyes half open, half close to see clear

THE BEAUTIFUL CURVE
Lift arms curved (with elbow fixed with arms as one unit) in "willow" position overhead, hands mark open and outward position. Caress space (palms outward) as you bring your arms down sideways, maintaining the beautiful curve, gracefully.

2. **ARMS**

a. **TORTOISE AND THE HARE**
(Move one hand slow the other faster U & D)
RUD - LCD, LUD - RCD x 3

b. **THE PARADOXICAL WINDMILL**
(Swing arms sideways F & B)
R initiates/L follows x 3
L initiates/R follows x3

c   **THE ROPE**
1. Push/pull rope to the front R push L pull,
Left push R pull x 10 each side
2. Parallel push U - D to squat, Rope pull up x 10

DO THE BEAUTIFUL CURVE

3. **HANDS**

a. **KNIFE-HANDS X 3 (straight lines movements)**
b. **HAND-ANGLES - Elbows D - Elbows U x 3**
c. **HANDULATIONS (Hands/Undulations)**

Hands together, x 3
R hand alone, L hand alone, x 3

d. **BALLS-CIRCLES/BOXES-SQUARES**
manipulate objects 3 sizes:
1. Object "smaller than me"
2. Object "like me"
3. Object "bigger than me"
Example:
1. **A Stone**, I can hold it,
2. **A Rock**, I can still move it
3. **A Mountain**, I walk on it

DO THE BEAUTIFUL CURVE

4. **STICKS**

a. FIST-MAKING ROUND x 1
b. FINGER REVOLUTIONS - F B x 3
c. FINGER TOSS F B x3
d. HAND TOSS
   1. one hand - RL x 3   2. Two x 6
   3. Lateral - RL, x 6   4. Vertical UD x 6

e. **COMPASS REFLECTION MOVEMENTS**
   1. with stick fixed at center through 8 points
      of compass X 1
   2. with stick overhead turning on axis R - x 3, L - x 3

DO THE BEAUTIFUL CURVE

5. **WALKS**

a. **PIVOTS** axis R x 3
b. **BASCULES**
to the side R-C- L x 6, F-C-B each leg x 3
c. **TOUR EIFFEL**
R-C-L/L-C-R x 6   F-C-B each leg x 3
d. **ELEMENTAL WALKS** 10 steps each
   1. Stone Walk   2. Wind Walk
   3. Fire Walk   4. Water Walk

DO THE BEAUTIFUL CURVE

e. **ANIMAL WALKS**
(4-step animal walk, alert response and pivot;
shift to 4-step human/animal walk for each)
1. Bear Walk   2. Cat Walk
3. Serpent "Walk"   4. Crane Walk

f. **WALK OF POWER/Aleph Walk** (10 steps)
(Embodying animal and human essences)

g. **WALK OF HUMANITY**
(Walk of Power in close group formations)

DO THE BEAUTIFUL CURVE

6. **MOVING BOX MEDITATION/Reflection Through Movement**

> Precious gift inside the box; move slowly, set down, and pick up. Contract and enlarge, transfer to one another, play with object, improvise and end with circling the square and squaring the circle

7. **GLOBE**

> **With your hands** hold a circle big as the globe, develop from large, six, then contract, small it, condense until you make it small and eat it as a pill. Play, improvise with various sizes. Practice circles, curves etc.

DO THE BEAUTIFUL CURVE

8. **SHAPE-SHIFTER-TOSS**   Alone or with partner, the tossed object becomes another object when received ! Example: Toss a ball and receive it as a box, Toss a stick and receive it as a sword etc. Improvise

THE INTEGRATIVE CYCLE

> Concludes in a calm, restful and contemplative state, or on a more active, playful note with shape shifter toss. After this cycle we are ready to begin exploring the ten basic components of **Body*Speak*™**. There are a few creative improvisational versions of this cycle, for beginners, advanced and professionals.

THE SELF-EVOLUTION CYCLE (4)

**Body*Speak*™ is a transformative art, a method of capturing the essence
of a movement or a state of being by a powerful process of identification.
A practical series of exercises to better your life & quicken your
Self-evolution process.**

**"If I am not for myself who is for me? and if I am only for myself who am I?
and if not NOW, when?."
Hillel**

**"You cannot teach a man anything, you can only help him find it within himself."
Galileo**

NOTES ON THE SELF-EVOLUTION CYCLE (4)

The detailed work of this cycle is not be published. You will learn it in its entirety after being introduced to **Body*Speak*™** training and acquiring a comprehensive understanding. Thus, this cycle is actually only transmitted privately to students who want to be involved deeply in this work, or to become practitioners of it. However, here is what to expect when mastering The Self-Evolution Cycle.

- Discover your dormant power to apply your talents for your benefit and others.
- Harness powerful techniques of non-verbal communication.
- Conquer seemingly complex principles in an easy way, with style and elegance.
- Learn to establish a rapport with yourself and your audience.
- Practice integration of the mind and body in a way that correlates with your daily projects.
- Create confidence through movement rather than meditation.
- Write your own life script, produce every scene, and lead in the role you love most.
- Play while learning and claim your own authority, avoiding external control, which is often deceptive.

LA SOURCE PUISSANTE

A Group of Exercises for Daily Practice

"Our power to be, to exist, to think, to act, to decide and make choices doesn't come from any outer source, it comes from the inner powerful source of our own individuality. This personal power doesn't come from our friends, teachers or parents. It springs from the inner creative source dynamically living within us. When we fully realize this individual power and awaken to this presence within, we become truly free, free to act, to think, to choose, to decide in a totally new dimension of being. With this new direction, the individual becomes creative and useful, helping others in the process to realize this power, to give more than one takes, to produce more than one consumes."

In a class session 1972

The La Source Puissante exercises are organized in 4 sections:

EXERCISE	Decribes the purpose of the practice.
MOVEMENT	Explains the physical movement of the practice.
TIME	Suggests how long and when to practice.
BENEFITS/RESULTS	Mentions a few benefits gained from the practice.

Please Note: Some of the exercises in this section may also be found in the "Creative Body*Speak*™ Exercise Sets" sections of this manual. Both versions are included to give a different contextual perspective on the exercises, with accompanying quotes that are also included in the "Anecdotes..." section of this Manual. As we will see, I like to take the "helicopter view," looking at the same subject from many angles.—Samuel

EXERCISE 1   STOP AND CONSIDER

Awareness of movement, continuous flow of activity, a practical tool to activate self-guidance and conscious thought, an attention-enhancing technique to sharpen the senses and extend the present moment.

MOVEMENT

Whatever movement you are doing at the time—walking washing dishes, cooking, running etc.—make a conscious decision to **Stop,** freeze the movement like a statue for few seconds, then continue the same movement in **Slow Motion** for a time and then back to your regular rhythm of movement. When you become natural at this, you can use this technique to **Reflect** on a specific thought or subject or make a decision you need at the time, and **Consider** the creativity of this very moment.

TIME

You can practice **Stop And Consider** anytime for 5 to 10 minutes. Do 5 or 10 sequences a day when possible. Be playful while doing it at home or when you are by yourself, or even teach it to your children. They probably will teach you a thing or two.

BENEFITS/RESULTS

- Stay awake and ready, aware of the present moment.
- Prevent accident, awkwardness, allow the flow of motion.
- Increase conscious thought and action; observe and allow change to occur.
- Master "**minimum movement, maximum expression.**"
- Enjoy a precious time to play and be with yourself.

Before the Word There Was Movement

"Movement is vibration, the essence of everything.
An intelligent being **thinks** and **talks**,
an emotional being **sings**,
an integrated being
thinks, talks, sings and moves...ACT."

EXERCISE 2   ONE DAY OF SILENCE:
Fast from words, Fast from food

In a world full of noise, it is suggested to choose one day a week and not use words to communicate. Simply practice silence, go about everyday activities, and observe your essential presence at work. You can choose half a day also, but do it regularly, the same day each week. Also, fasting one day from foods, once every 2 weeks will regenerate your digestive system and allow it to rest.

MOVEMENT

Every moment of your day of silence will be filled with special awareness and new challenges. How you do things—as you sit, stand, eat, or any activity—will be of great significance.

TIME

Establish a specific day and stick to it regularly.

BENEFITS/RESULTS
- Develop a keen sense of self-observation.
- Achieve calmness, poise and tranquility.
- Use your time effectively and economically.
- Become both calm and energetic by practicing word economy.
- Speak less and do more; your activity will have meaning and usefulness.
- Become aware of every little movement and realize the power of the word.

Word Economy

My grandfather once told me that we are born with a certain number of words in our **word bank**. If we use too many words (like checks or spending too much) and empty the word bank, we might become overdrawn, or mute. When necessary, words are one of the ways to communicate; 90% of our real communication, however, occurs in silence, through body language.

"I highly recommend using silence and awareness to speak less
and do more and produce more and consume less
— practicing consistently the wisdom of the word economy."

55

EXERCISE 3   FIRST THOUGHT, LAST THOUGHT (FTLT)

Become aware of your first thought when you awake in the morning and your last thought before you sleep. Before you sleep, do a **daily review** of your thoughts and experiences of the day and resolve to sleep well with a clean conscience of having lived that day with awareness and honesty.

MOVEMENT

While in bed before awakening and in while going to sleep.

TIME

Before you sleep and when you awake.

BENEFITS/RESULTS

- Awaken genuine awareness of your thoughts and the way you function.
- Be able to make decisions clearly and productively.
- Discover and explore the source of thinking and who is the thinker .
- Develop creative writing as a tool for observing the change and activate the poet within you.

Hear, See, Do and Understand

Consider this nugget of wisdom:
"When I hear, I forget. When I see, I remember. When I do, I understand."
So, if you really want to really learn and know, **Do, Act.**
Knowledge without action is **utterly worthless.**
Wouldn't you agree?."

EXERCISE 4   ARTISTIC ZERO

Artistic Zero is a physically, mentally and emotionally balanced posture of alertness and calm readiness. A place, a center of silence and poise where you can choose where to go, this way or that way. A state where you are present every moment you breathe. A place of orientation that swells from the "Presence Zone". Artistic Zero is also a way to bond with gravity.

MOVEMENT

To practice Artistic Zero, position yourself with your back to the wall. Visualize a plumb line going from the top of your head to your heels. Stay still, breathe comfortably. Feel yourself lift vertically in balance against the wall. The body is learning to deal with the gravity of the moment.

Do the same posture horizontally while lying on your back and relaxing. In both vertical and horizontal positions become aware of yourself where you are and just breathe calmly.

TIME

Consciously do this 3 times a day, 5 minutes each time.

BENEFITS/RESULTS
- Achieve a sense of who you are and where are you now.
- Become aware of erect posture, gravity, balance.
- Digest your food better
- Breathe easier allowing your organism to fulfill its natural function
- Change your posture to change the way you think, be, and act
- Feel yourself moving within the current of life

REMEMBER and REALIZE

Identify and eliminate laziness and dishonesty in yourself and live passionately without guilt. Be always ready, alert, and responsive to the beautiful and vibrant life within you. Happiness is your natural state. It does not depend on anyone but your own self. Enjoy every present moment of your life. Remember! Your life is your moment in eternity. It is precious and can be full of joy.

EXERCISE 5   **THE PRESENCE ZONE: The Posture of Enchantment, or The Turnkey Posture**

This Presence Zone practice is closely connected with the practice of the Artistic Zero. The idea is to integrate the two in order to sense the power within yourself.

MOVEMENT   For this practice you are free to choose any comfortable movement. You can sit, walk or stand, lean against a tree. Notice your calm breathing. Just watch your thoughts passing through, like birds flying. Observe them from this state. Let them go and just be.

TIME   Consciously do this 3 times a day, 5 minutes each time.

BENEFITS/RESULTS
- Be complete unto yourself, present every moment, on your own
- Increase your joy of awareness of who you are at this present moment

Seize The Day, Shape The Space

When you practice the Presence Zone exercise you accomplish what I call "elasticizing time and space." You can choose to live totally. There are no excuses.

EXERCISE 6   ONE DAILY MINUTE OF LAUGHTER

This practice will release all body/mind tensions introducing a joyous state. Laugh out of existence all thoughts, emotions and situations that are not good for you and that block your way.

MOVEMENT

Stand before the mirror, place your hand on your hips, bend the knees slightly, look at yourself, and laugh while shaking the body up and down. Watching yourself laugh even more vigorously. Laugh from the diaphragm not the throat. Be aware of your jaws and release tension by dropping your jaw slightly.

TIME

Consciously do this 3 times a day, 5 minutes each time. Do in the morning upon awakening or whenever you feel yourself upset or frustrated. You may realize a deep sense of sadness. Enjoy your sadness.

BENEFITS/RESULTS
- Discover areas of your body never used before.
- Release tensions from various areas of the body.
- Increase silliness; we have lost the power of silliness.
- Shake your whole body and spirit to live more passionately.

Who is leading your life?

Who is writing your script? Be the author and lead actor in your life—now.
Unleash the fearless creative power within you.
I am not a human **being**, I am a human **becoming**.

EXERCISE 7   RESPOND vs. REACT

Responding is voluntary; reacting is not voluntary. Responding comes from balance and attention; reacting comes from fear and distraction. Reacting is hazardous to your health.

MOVEMENT

Wherever you are—having a conversation, answering a question—take time to take a breath in silence before you respond. When you talk, speak calmly by choice. Breathe your words.

TIME

Consciously do this 3 times a day, 5 minutes each time until it become your natural way to respond.

BENEFITS/RESULTS

- Let go of automatic behavior.
- Observe the newness of things.
- Increase your sense of your own value.
- Achieve gentleness with yourself and others.
- Live and let live, with increased appreciation of life.

What is a Genuine Being ?

Not every guitar-scratcher is a musician,
Not every white face in Town Square is a mime or clown,
Not every house painter is a Picasso,
Not every menu writer is a poet.

EXERCISE 8   UNE CHOSE à LA FOIS, One Thing At A Time

MOVEMENT   Focus on one thing at a time as if it is done for the first and last time. Break down into small movements or actions the components of the task or project to finish in less time than a scattered mind would take. Attend to the action at the time of the action. This practice goes hand-in-hand with "From Ecstasy to Lunch."

TIME   Consciously do this 3 times a day, 5 minutes each time until it is established as a consistent state of being.

BENEFITS/RESULTS
- Master "minimum effort, maximum result."
- Finish projects in a shorter time than usual.
- Direct conscious effort to fulfilling your dreams and desires.
- Eliminate procrastination and laziness, boredom and anxiety.
- Increase the ability to concentrate and achieve rapidly in all areas of life.

This Precious Moment

"Thought is the blossom; language the bud; action is the fruit behind it."
"This time, like all times, is a very good time if we but know what to do
…that is genius."

Ralph Waldo Emerson

EXERCISE 9   "FROM ECSTASY TO LUNCH"

The power to SHIFT your attention from this to that, this state to that state, from the sublime to the practical, from thought to action, from this action to the next action, always present, will make you more physically and mentally agile. Shift easily from here to there at will without awkwardness or accidents or any emotional upsets, able overcome all interruptions and remaining focused from moment to moment.

MOVEMENT

While doing any activity, sharply stop the flow of that activity. Do something else for a short while, then stop again and go to the next action. Shift attention quickly. Do this with focused awareness. Do not be hectic. Be mindful as you train yourself to develop this skill.

TIME

Consciously do this 3 times a day, 5 minutes each time until it is established as a consistent practice.

BENEFITS/RESULTS
- Use your attention effectively.
- Increase your intelligence and memory.
- Discover the process of learning how to learn.
- Reduce worries and use stress to serve your accomplishment of the task.
- Use time properly with less movement while performing a task, so it takes 30 minutes to do what everyone does in 5 hours.

"La Pensée vol, Les mots vont à pied." - "Thoughts fly, words walk."

Etienne Decroux

"Nothing in life is to be feared, it is only to be understood."

Madame Marie Curie

EXERCISE 10   **"THE VIEW FROM THE HELICOPTER AND THE BOAT"**

The ability to see things as they are from two levels: the objective (the helicopter-whole) and the subjective (the boat-details) to integrate and see the whole. From the boat, your view is personal, limited, with blinders; from the helicopter, you can see the whole from different angles. Making decisions after exploring both ways of seeing will be beneficial.

MOVEMENT   Relax your body in any position you choose while seeing yourself AS IF you are in the helicopter or the boat.

TIME   Consciously do this 3 times a day, 5 minutes each time until it is established as a consistent state of being.

BENEFITS/RESULTS
- Be 100% involved in life.
- Integrate subjective and objective realities.
- Make a leap to dare to think what others do not yet imagine.
- Discover new ways of seeing, perceiving and conceptualizing.
- Surprise yourself with these two ways of viewing the universe.

Helio+Geo-Centric Integrated View of Reality

"Body*Speak*™ is **not** psychotherapy. It sprang from an artistic view of the universe, an integrated view of reality (boat + helicopter, right + left cerebral hemispheres, sun + earth centric). It is creatively oriented to identify the inconsistencies between your thoughts and actions. It restores your natural balance, aligning your expression, speech and movements. Body*Speak*™ is a transformative art, a method of capturing the essence of a movement or a state of being by a powerful process of identification and integration."

CREATIVE Body*Speak*™ EXERCISES

Please Note: A few of the exercises in this section have been adapted to the Four Longevity Cycles. They complement and elaborate certain details in the exercises presented here to improve the vibrant health of the body.—Samuel

OUTLINE

Creative Body*Speak*™ Exercise Set 1: CREATIVE MENTALITY

1. The View from the BOAT and the HELICOPTER
2. The IMPERMEABLE
3. Seventy-five -Twenty five - 75/25
4. Stop and Consider
5. Patterns of Movement: "Making a MAP of your day"
6. The ELAN
7. The EYE COMPASS Exercise
8. The British Flag
9. S.A.F.A = Shift Attention - Focus Attention

Creative Body*Speak*™ Exercise Set 2: ARTISTIC ZERO

1. Artistic Zero
2. Spiral Drops
3. Postures
4. Space Awareness
5. Willow Tree
6. Turnkey Posture or The Posture of Enchantment

Creative Body*Speak*™ Exercise Set 3: THE STRETCH EXERCISES

1. Leg Stretches
2. The Tiger
3. Rock Climbing
4. The Door knob
5. Wall Stretch, side to side
6. Chair Spine Stretch
7. The "L" Leg Stretch
8. The "I" Stretch

Creative Body*Speak*™ Exercise Set 4: SITTING POSTURE

The Egyptian Posture

Creative Body*Speak*™ Exercise Set 5: VERTICAL EXERCISE SERIES

      1. Wall Arm Sweeps
      2. Vertical Wall Squats
      3. Vertical Squats
      4. Pelvic Work

Creative Body*Speak*™ Exercise Set 6: HORIZONTAL EXERCISE SERIES

      1. Spinal Stretch
      2. Weight Lifting
      3. Floor Arms Sweeps

Creative Body*Speak*™ Exercise Set 7: HAND EXERCIES – L'ORIENTALE – 1-6

Creative Body*Speak*™ Exercise Set 8: ARM EXERCISES

      1. Wrists Shaking
      2. Windmill Pattern

Creative Body*Speak*™ Exercise Set 9: BASIC HANDS EXPRESSIONS

      1. Basic Hands Exercise
      2. So What?
      3. L'Orientale 1-6
      4. The Beautiful
      5. The Apple
      6. The Ball
      7. Flat Hand Knife Exercise
      8. Defining a Box
      9. The Moving Box – Slow motion reflection
      10. The Globe
      11. Pointing the Finger
      12. Plate Turning
      13. Objects, Variations, Etudes

Creative Body*Speak*™ Exercise Set 1

CREATIVE MENTALITY

1. **THE VIEW FROM THE BOAT AND THE HELICOPTER**
2. **The IMPERMEABLE**
3. **SEVENTY-FIVE-TWENTY-FIVE- 75/25**
4. **STOP AND CONSIDER**
5. **PATTERNS OF MOVEMENT: "MAKING MAP OF YOUR D A Y "**
6. **THE ELAN**
7. **THE EYE COMPASS EXERCISE**
8. **THE BRITISH FLAG**
9. **S.A.F.A = SHIFT ATTENTION – FOCUS ATTENTION**

These exercises were designed to address certain aspects of mental attitude, to enhance and activate creative thinking, opening new ways of learning to organize and increase conscious awareness, enhance physical work of the body, and overcome any presently limiting mindset.

1. The View from the BOAT and the HELICOPTER

Exercise: This exercise asks you to take a view of things you do daily in life as if you were in a boat, and then, view your situation as if you were in a helicopter. This is a good exercise to do before making new and important decisions in all aspects of your life.

Definition: The view from **the boat** is limited. Here we view our own "individual" little worlds. We learn how we contain, confine, and restrict ourselves in space and in various situations. It's like wearing horse blinders. We can ask questions such as: What makes me think and act the way I do? What steps did I take to carry out necessary actions? Did I waste time and energy doing these actions?

In the boat we can be aware of how "busy" we are with the details of life. We can observe our emotional reactions to the "dramas" which sometimes lead to irrational thinking and sloppy doing. This is a **subjective** view.

The view from the **helicopter** is unlimited. In the helicopter, one views the self as if from the ceiling. From this objective perch, we can look beyond the physical body. Here, one can expand their way of thinking, move beyond the physical limitations of the self, take a clear perspective of the situation and think creatively. Because this is an objective view, interest lies more for the good of all rather than just for the individual.

Key words for the view from the boat and from the helicopter:

Boat	Helicopter
Limited	Unlimited
For the separate self	The good of all (the whole)
Details	Whole picture
The physical body	Non-physical (spiritual)
Confined	Free
Containment	Openness, spaciousness, expanded
Emotions	Creative Mentality
Irrational (at times)	Rational (most of the time)
Subjective	Objective

Benefits: Integrate your way of seeing, thinking, and acting in balance, both physical and mental dimensions.
Function from a calm state and be able to make rational decisions. think and act clearly without harming anyone or anything.
See details in the whole, and the whole in the details, thus living 100%.

2. The IMPERMEABLE

Definition: A practical mental state that does not allow events to affect one's balance and harmony. The ability to be involved, yet remain detached and objective.

Exercise: Visualize a raincoat with the rain drops sliding over the surface leaving a trace of water, keeping the surface dry. The water of the rain does not affect the surface of the coat.

Benefits: Learn to become calmly detached, but not indifferent to interacting with the world.

3. SEVENTY-FIVE/TWENTY-FIVE - 75/25

Definition: This is a good mental exercise for considering how we utilize awareness in our everyday life. Seventy-five percent (75%) is the executor (the body), the one who carries out the actions. Twenty-five percent (25%) is the director (the mind), the one who observes the actor in life.

75/25 is a state of being aware of both thinking and doing simultaneously. 75/25 is an exercise for learning to narrow the gap between thought and action. To activate oneself into doing more.

Exercise: This exercise asks you to be aware of the thinker and the doer for one moment, one hour, or even one day. To be aware of what you think and how much you talk, versus how much you actually do with what you think.

Benefits: Balance thinking and doing for accurate decision making.
Increase awareness of how you think and do.

Reduce and eliminates procrastination and laziness in life, and to accomplish more in less time.

4. STOP AND CONSIDER

Definition: In this exercise, you are asked to be aware of unnecessary movements you do everyday, movements that waste time and energy. Have you ever stopped to consider how many movements it takes you to perform a daily activity?

Exercise: Take one activity such as drinking a glass of water, getting ready for work, eating, or any other activity in the process of being done. Try to be aware of every movement your body makes for that whole activity (fingers, hands, wrists, elbows, legs, etc.). Count the movements.

Example: Go into the kitchen to drink a glass of water. As you go to the kitchen at your regular pace, **STOP** yourself in place. Do not move. Think about just walking into the kitchen.

Now, walk to the kitchen in **slow motion**. **Slowly** take a glass of water. Fill the glass of water. **Slowly** drink from the glass of water. Very **slowly** place the glass on the counter. Now walking at your regular pace, go back to the living room or other area of the home and continue with your regular activity.

Now try this with other activities. Stop and consider your activity in slow motion and then at regular speed.

Benefits: The more you master this exercise, the easier you will achieve **"minimum movement, maximum expression**, and **"minimum effort, maximum results."** As a result, you can achieve in a short period of time what used to take you a long time.

5. PATTERNS OF MOVEMENT: "MAKING A MAP OF YOUR DAY"

Definition: Observe the patterns of movement you make room-to-room, place-to-place for one day. Notice how your day takes shape.

Exercise: Draw a map of your daily activities from the moment you wake up until you go to sleep at night. Write down every activity in detail. Draw every movement of the day right after you do it. (For example, if you travel from the house to the food store, draw a series of lines representing the road from your house to the store and through the food store and back home again, etc.

See former student Steve Rusan's illustration and description of this exercise in *Mime & Beyond - The Silent Outcry*, p.102.

Benefits: Keep awake, alert and ready and stay open to the present moment.
Begin to become consciously aware of unnecessary movements made and how you could eliminate them and conserve energy.

6. THE ELAN

Definition: A mental attitude to activate the dynamism, energy and power of movement. The spring before the action. The propulsive force behind the action. Joy and enthusiasm for what you are doing, the passage from the technical to the spontaneous, enthusiastic, vigorous, and lively, with a distinctive style and flair, maintaining momentum.

Example:
1. Before you step forward, you prepare with a step backward.
2. Before you throw the discus, you turn back before propelling forward.
3. Before leaping forward, you crouch back.

Benefits: Achieve the harmonious distribution and circulation of energy to appreciate your existence.

7. The EYE COMPASS EXERCISE

Definition: Eye movement coordination exercise (see following page).

Benefits: Increase focus and concentration.
Calm and center your nervous system.
Enhance visual memory recall.

Note: When this eye exercise is done daily, your whole being begins to function from a calm state. Observe how your thoughts and movements become serene in the midst of activity. Observe how your breathing becomes calmer after finishing these eye exercises.

THE EYE COMPASS™:
A special exercise of the Body*Speak*™ method
benefiting one's orientation, direction, and decisions.

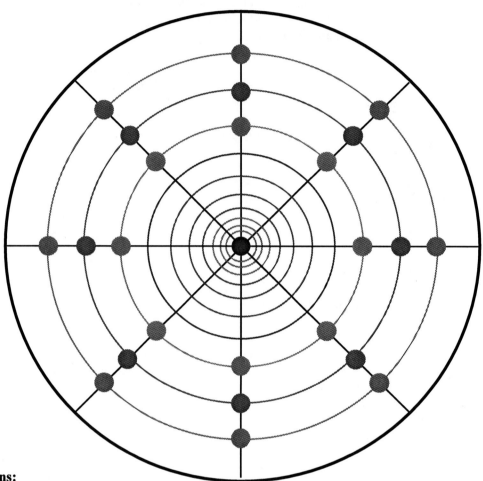

Directions:

1. Focus on the **center dot**.

2. Follow the **smallest ring**, the one closest to the center dot outward six times clockwise and then counter-clockwise with your eyes. Repeat for each ring from **smallest to largest**.

3. Next, follow **the first circle of dots** after the rings, which we will call **the inner circle**. Stop the eye movement at each dot and focus on the spot. Then, follow six times clockwise and then counter-clockwise. Repeat with **the middle circle** and then **the outer circle**.

4. Finally, follow **the outermost circle** with your eye six times clockwise and then six times counter-clockwise.

8. THE BRITISH FLAG

Description: The four (4) basic eye position movements are:

1. Lateral left, center focus, lateral right (side-side).
2. Upper central, center focus, lower central (up/down).
3. Upper left, center focus, lower right (diagonal).
4. Upper right, center focus, lower left (diagonal).

British Flag - Exercise. Set I

1. Sit or stand relaxed. Begin with eyes centrally focused and relaxed.
2. Move eyes sharply to lateral left. Stay. Return to central focus.
3. Move eyes sharply to lateral right. Stay. Return to central focus.

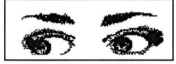 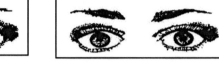 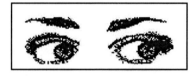

| **Lateral Right** | **Central Focus** | **Lateral left** |

British Flag - Exercise. Set II

1. Begin with eyes centrally focused and relaxed.
2. Move eyes sharply to upper central. Stay. Return to central focus.
3. Move eyes sharply to lower central. Stay. Return to central focus.

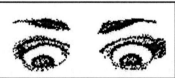 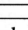 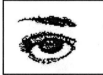

| **Lower Central** | **Central Focus** | **Upper Central** |

British Flag - Exercise. Set III

1.   Begin with eyes centrally focused and relaxed.
2.   Move eyes sharply to upper left. Stay. Return to central focus.
3.   Move eyes sharply to lower right. Stay. Return to central focus.

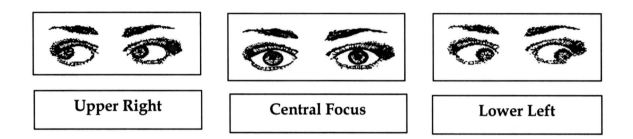

Upper Right   **Central Focus**   **Lower Left**

British Flag - Exercise. Set IV

1.   Begin with eyes centrally focused and relaxed.
2.   Move eyes sharply to upper right. Stay. Return to central focus.
3.   Move eyes sharply to lower left. Stay. Return to central focus.

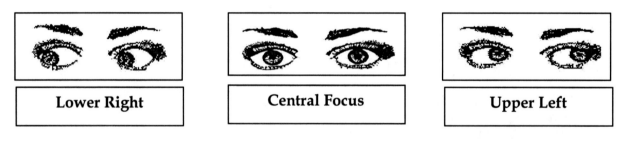

Lower Right   **Central Focus**   **Upper Left**

Note: Do all four sets three times. Raise the lids while doing the down sets of the eye exercises. Don't raise your eyebrows.

EYE ROLLS

Right eye rolls - Start at central focus, move the eyes to lateral left, then, upper left, upper central, upper right, lateral right, lower right, lower central, lower left, lateral left, and then back to central focus. Relax the eyes.

Left eye rolls - Start at central focus, move the eyes to lateral right, then, upper right, upper central, upper, left, lateral left, lower left, lower central, lower right, lateral right and then back to central focus. Relax the eyes. **Do three sets of each.**

9.   S.A.F.A = SHIFT ATTENTION – FOCUS ATTENTION

Definition: The basic tool to use for attention is the eyes. Generally, eye movements are unconscious, awareness slippery and fluffy. Once we master the discipline of **SAFA**, we can change the way we think by visualizing with clarity.

Exercise: Sit quietly and comfortably, and place your right hand before you, look at the palm and place your attention on each of your fingers, one by one. Observe the lines, texture, colors and various marks.
Take 5 breaths for each finger. Pay attention to each phalange and the space between the fingers. Then shift gently to the next finger, until you finish all your fingers.

Now, look at the whole hand, and observe where your attention is, on what finger, and how long your attention stays there until it is shifted, just observe your eye movements and relax.

Now repeat the same with the other hand, and relax your eyes. Also practice the EYE COMPASS exercise from the Flexibility Cycle, to get used to these eye movements.

Benefits: You will master this simple technique and develop your own way to improvise.

You can create new ways to use your attention. Shift attention, focus attention on an object, event, image, color, or person.
Observe yourself doing the exercise. Then choose a specific area of attention, an event or a thought, and work on it until you feel at ease with the process.

Example: Now take another subject, topic or goal and repeat the whole process again. If you get bored, it is s good sign, but you must graduate "boredom" to go beyond objects, events and persons. You can now take any project and work it the same way, and enjoy its manifestation. While you are at it, observe kindly how many things about your behavior have changed from what was sloppy to what now is excellent and focused.

Creative Body*Speak*™ Exercise Set 2

CREATIVE INTEGRATED CONCEPTS

1. ARTISTIC ZERO
2. SPIRAL DROPS
3. POSTURES
4. SPACE AWARENESS
5. WILLOW TREE
6. POSTURE
   OR THE POSTURE OF ENCHANTMENT
   OR THE TURNKEY POSTURE

Exercises to integrate the mental image of the exercise with the physical practice. These are also general instructions for how to use various parts of the body and activate whole body movement.

1. ARTISTIC ZERO

Definition: Artistic zero is a mental and physical vertical posture where one is in a state of readiness or to which one returns to re-set the body and mind after an activity. A center from which one move in any direction. A center from which one can orient oneself.

Exercise:
1. Stand with feet in first position.
2. Relax arms at sides. Eyes should focus on the horizon.
3. Relax, sense the circulation of the breath throughout the body.
4. Think of your spine as a vertical line running from the bottom of your feet through the top of your head.
5. Remain very still and breathe. Hold this posture in a relaxed state while circulating the breath for approximately 2-5 minutes.

Benefits: Increase focus and concentration.
Calm and still the inner being.
Become aware of motion in stillness.

2. SPIRAL DROPS

Exercise: Stand in the center of the room. Relax. In a gracefully spiraling motion, drop from vertical to horizontal until you are lying down on the floor. Do it in slow motion first, and then at natural speed.
Do three turns each direction, right and left.

Benefits: Release physical and mental tension.
Achieve fearlessness in falling.

3. POSTURES

Exercise:
1. Choose five different postures.
2. Create the first posture. Keep still.
3. Breathe quietly. Count the number of breaths.
4. Focus the eyes on a specific point, then slowly shift to the next posture.
5. Continue this pattern until you have done all five postures.

Hold each posture 2-5 minutes.

Benefits:
Increase focus, concentration and the ability to center.
Increase physical and mental endurance.

3. SPACE AWARENESS

Exercise:
Stand in Artistic Zero.
1. Walk forward, backward, side-to-side in a straight line with eyes open. Repeat with eyes closed.
2. Walk a perfect circle forward from left to right and then backward, right to left. Do this with eyes open. Repeat this sequence with eyes closed.
3. Walk a triangle, square, and rectangle, forward and backward with eyes open. Repeat this sequence with eyes closed.

Benefits:
Develop internal balance, equilibrium and spatial awareness for inner and outer orientation.

4. WILLOW TREE

Exercise:
1. Stand in Artistic Zero.
2. Raise arms above the head.
3. Relax the elbows.
4. Allow the wrists to drop like a willow tree.
5. Hold the posture for 2-5 minutes.
6. Breathe slowly, calm and relaxed. When time is up, bring the hands slowly down, caressing the space.
7. Relax and repeat this exercise a few times to tolerance level.

Benefits:
Releases body tension.
Enhances calm, peacefulness and stillness in the body.

5. TURNKEY POSTURE

Exercise:
Begin with Artistic Zero.
Choose a posture. Maintain that posture for five minutes.
Work up to 10 minutes. Remember to tense, breathe, release when you are in posture.

Samuel Avital

Benefits: Increase focus, concentration and stillness of the being.
Daydream and plan more creatively.
Better visualize a specific outcome.

76

Creative Body*Speak*™ Exercise Set 3

THE STRETCH EXERCISES

1. **LEG STRETCHES**
2. **THE TIGER**
3. **ROCK CLIMBING**
4. **THE DOORKNOB**
5. **WALL STRETCH SIDE TO SIDE**
6. **CHAIR SPINE STRETCH**
7. **The "L" LEG STRETCH**
8. **The "I" STRETCH**

1. LEG STRETCHES

Stand with legs slightly apart. Bend over. Plant hands palm side down on the ground. Bring one leg forward. Put the other leg back. Bend forward leg while straightening and stretching the back leg. Do five stretches with each leg, then switch legs.

2. THE TIGER

This can be done on the floor or up the stairs. Get on all fours.
While moving forward, stretch a front limb forward and out, while at the same time, stretching the opposite leg backwards and out. Then do the opposite side. Do while crawling forward.

3. ROCK CLIMBING

Lie on the floor face down. Use your arms and legs. Pretend you are climbing a rock face.

4. THE DOOR KNOB

1. **Side Stretch** - Stand sideways to a door. Hold the door with your hand. Stretch your right hand at arm's length. Bend the right knee. Stretch the left leg as far as you can in the opposite direction. Stretch the left arm over your head as you stretch outward with the left leg. Keep the body straight during the side inclination. Switch and do the left hand holding the door and do the right arm over the head, stretching while the right leg is stretching outward and back.
2. **Front Stretch** - Face the door. At arm's length, hold the doorknob with the right hand. Bend the right knee. Stretch the left leg back maintaining a straight leg and a straight diagonal inclination. Keep the left arm hanging down towards the floor. The head should be looking toward the floor. Switch and do the left hand and right leg stretching outward.
3. **Front Stretch** (legs together) - Face the door. Grasp the doorknob with both hands. Maintain feet in first position. Take a breath in. Then, <u>slowly</u> exhale

77

while being conscious of stretching the spine while <u>slowly</u> bending forward at the waist until the trunk is horizontal with the arms. Pause for fifteen seconds. Then, <u>slowly</u> ascend to a standing position while inhaling with movement originating from the pelvis. Be aware of each vertebra when coming up.

5. WALL STRETCH - SIDE TO SIDE

Exercise: Stand against a wall. Place the feet in second position. Pretend that you are a sandwich. Vertebra by vertebra starting with the head, bend toward the right side while maintaining the position against the wall (side inclination). Bend the trunk as far as you can to the side. Once you are bent all the way over to the side, shift the pelvis to that side. Then begin with the head and repeat the above exercise moving toward the left side.

Repeat this exercise three times in each direction.

Benefits: Isolate each vertebra.
Make the spine more supple and flexible.
Increase lung capacity. Oxygenate the lower parts of the lungs.

6. CHAIR SPINE STRETCH

Exercise: Put a chair in front of you at arm's length. Bend at the waist and hold onto the chair with your hands. Put the right leg out in front while keeping the left leg in neutral position. Bend the knees. While pushing the chair straight forward with the arms, focus on extending the spine, vertebra by vertebra.   Go to full extension. Exhale the breath while moving toward extension. Hold full extension for 15 seconds. Slowly while inhaling draw the chair back while returning to the neutral position of standing and fully exhale. Repeat the exercise on the other side.
Do this five times on each side.

Benefit: Make the spine more supple and flexible.

7. THE "L" LEG STRETCH

Exercise: Lie on the floor. Bring buttocks to the wall. Put legs straight in the air against the wall. There should be no space between the wall and the body. Hold for five minutes or longer.

8. THE "I" SPINE STRETCH

Exercise: Stand against the wall. Place feet in first position. Use a stick to support movement down and forward. Place the stick to the side and in front of the body. Hold the stick with the right hand.   Try to bend all the way forward vertebra by vertebra until the head almost touches the knees. Try to keep the pelvis in contact

with the wall. The hand movement on the stick should coordinate with each isolated vertebra movement. Slowly go back to standing position. Remember to breathe. Repeat and do on the left side.
Do this exercise three times on each side.

Benefit: Isolate the vertebrae and make the spine supple.

Creative Body*Speak*™ Exercise Set 4

SITTING POSTURE

EGYPTIAN POSTURE

Exercise: Sit in chair with spine erect. Plant feet firmly on the floor. Legs should be 1-2 fists apart with thighs straight toward the horizon. Measure distance between the knees. Rest hands on lap, palms down. Relax hands. Look straight ahead. Eyes on the horizon. Find one point to focus on. Maintain this posture for five minutes. Be conscious of the breath.

Benefit: Increase focus, concentration and maintain stillness of the being.

EGYPTIAN POSTURE IN FIVE (5) MOVEMENTS

Instruction:

1. **Shoulder Height** - Sit in a chair with spine erect. Plant feet firmly on the floor. Legs should be 1-2 fists apart with thighs straight toward the horizon. Measure distance between the knees. Rest arms and hands straight down at sides. Slowly sweep arms up (palm-side down) to **shoulder height**. Keep wrist bent and fingers together with hands and elbows relaxed while coming up. Maintain this posture for approximately five minutes. Increase the holding time of this position. Be aware of the breath.

2. **Willow Tree Arms** - After maintaining the posture at shoulder height, sweep the arms up overhead, maintaining wrists bent, palms down. Turn fingers of both hands toward each other. Elbows should be slightly relaxed. Hold arms up overhead in this position for five minutes. Like a willow tree.

3. **Eagle Spread** - From the willow tree, sweep the arms down slowly with hands palm-side out caressing the space until hands at about a 45° angle. Arms and hands should become a straight line. Fingers together. Maintain this posture for five minutes. Then, bring hands and arms down to side in a slow sweep, caressing the space.

4. **Completion (TBR - tense, breathe, release)**

   a. Sit in Egyptian posture. Make a fist with thumbs inside of fist. Place them on your thighs. Inhale and hold the breath. Slowly begin to tense the fists. Next tense the lower arms, then the upper arms, shoulders, chest, abdomen, thighs, knees, lower legs, and feet. Press the feet as if into the floor. Hold tension for five seconds. Release with a vigorous exhalation while maintaining form and then, slowly relax all the muscles.

   b. Next, press the feet into the floor. Tense the neck, jaw, teeth, cheek bones, nose, eyes, forehead and the skull. Hold tension for five seconds.

Release with a vigorous exhalation while maintaining form and then, slowly relax all the muscles.

c.   While pressing the feet into the floor, tense the feet, calves, knees, thighs, pelvis, abdomen, chest, shoulders, upper and lower arms, and hands. Hold tension for five seconds. Release with a vigorous exhalation while maintaining form and then slowly relax all the muscles.

5.   Repeat **The Egyptian Posture** to complete the cycle.

Note: The mind should focus on each individual body part while working through the various series of tension.

The Benefits: Calm the nervous system.
Increase inner silence.
Prepare for contemplation and decision making.
Be in close touch with each individual body part, mentally and physically.

Creative Body*Speak*™ Exercise Set 5

VERTICAL EXERCISE SERIES

> 1. WALL ARM SWEEPS
> 2. VERTICAL WALL SQUATS
> 3. VERTICAL SQUATS
> 4. PELVIC WORK

1. WALL ARM SWEEPS

Exercise: Stand against the wall. Maintain verticality. Have arms at sides with palms facing the wall. Slowly sweep the arms up overhead while maintaining contact with the wall. Turn palms over when it feels natural as the arms rise. Inhale as the arms ascend. Hold for 10-15 seconds. Exhale fully. Inhale again, then slowly sweep arms down to neutral position. **Do five times.**

Benefit: Increase lung capacity.

2. VERTICAL WALL SQUATS

Exercise: Stand against the wall. Keep the whole spine straight. Exhale slowly and lower the self to a squatting position without the body leaving the wall. Maintain verticality. Spread the feet far enough apart to support the weight of the body. Slowly lower the body to a squatting position. Exhale as you go down. Hold for 10-15 seconds. Then, go from the squatting to the standing position, slowly inhaling as you rise. Lead with the head. Upward movement should be from the pelvis. Maintain verticality while going up. Fully exhale and relax all muscles. **Do five times.**

Benefit: Enhance circulation of the life force.
Increase strength and endurance of the spine and legs.

3. VERTICAL SQUATS

Exercise: Stand in the center of the room. Do the above exercise without the support of the wall. Maintain verticality and breathe.

Benefit: Increase strength and endurance of the spine and legs.

4. PELVIC WORK

1. Double Pin   Find Artistic Zero. Then, find a good stance with legs slightly apart, knees bent. Imagine the thumb as a pin. Imagine the pin going right below your belly button with the pelvis going backward. The pin then pushes the pelvis forward at the sacrum. Do five double pin movements without moving the rest of the body.

2. Pelvic Isolations

Stand with legs apart. Bend the knees. Move the pelvis sharply backward, forward, side-side. **Do five times in each direction.**

Benefit: Circulate life force.
Lubricate pelvis and hip joints.
Learnto stabilize and balance postures.

Creative BodySpeak™ Exercise Set 6

HORIZONTAL EXERCISE SERIES

1. **SPINAL STRETCH**
2. **WEIGHT LIFTING**
3. **FLOOR ARM SWEEPS**

1. SPINAL STRETCH

Exercise: Lie on the floor on your back. Beginning with the pelvis, lead to the left side vertebra by vertebra. Do not move the extremities or head until it is its turn to lead. Move from the pelvis to the top of the head. Turn until you are prone. Roll back and do the other side. Next, from the prone position, lead with the pelvis. Vertebra by vertebra turn from the belly onto the back. **Do this exercise three times very slowly.**

Benefit: Increase flexibility and suppleness of the spine.

2. WEIGHT SHIFTING

Exercise: Lie face down on the floor. Put arms out in front of the body above the head. Palms down. Sweep arms back to shoulder level. Bend elbows, plant palms of hands on floor. Have pelvis lead up and backward to bent knee position. Bring right leg up, plant foot on floor. Shift weight to right side. Bring left leg up, plant foot on floor. Center weight over pelvis. Exhale. Then while inhaling, slowly rise to standing position from the squatting position. Exhale and relax. **Do this exercise three times very slowly.**

Benefit: Develop conscious awareness of each movement.

3. FLOOR ARM SWEEPS

Exercise: Lie on floor. Arms at side. Palms face down. Slowly sweep arms up over top of head while maintaining contact with the floor at all times. Inhale while ascending. Exhale when arms reach above head. Pause for 10-15 seconds. Inhale, then turn palms over and sweep the arms slowly back down to sides while exhaling and maintaining contact with the floor at all times. **Do this exercise three times very slowly.**

Benefit: Relax trunk and arms.

Creative Body*Speak*™ Exercise Set 7

HAND EXERCISES – L'ORIENTALE – 1-6

1.   Place the palms of your two hands together with the fingers touching - two hands as one.

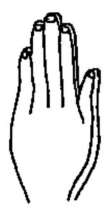

2.   Spread the fingers wide apart, keeping the fingers and palm of one hand fully in contact with the fingers and palm of the other.

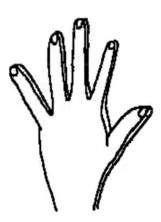

3.   Move the hands from position in 2, so that the fingertips and the base of the palms are touching as though one were holding a perfect ball.

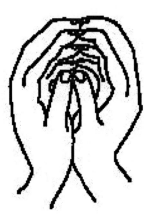

4.   Keeping the fingertips of the left hand together with the fingertips of the right hand, bring the palms of both hands together so that they are flat and touching. Do this in one count, quickly.

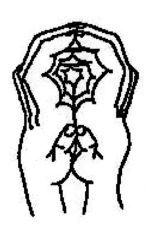

5.   Slowly raise the fingers as though a string were attached to the fingertips pulling them skyward so that the fingers and palm of one hand are flat against the fingers and palm of the other.

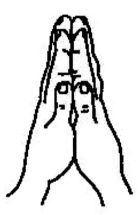

6.   Gradually peel back the fingers toward the back of the hand, keeping the palms touching. Slowly return to position one. After doing the series (1-6) times, shake out the hands vigorously and relax them.

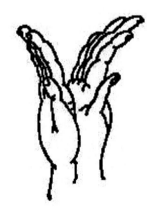

C r e a t i v e   B o d y *S p e a k* ™   E x e r c i s e   S e t   8

HAND EXERCISES continued

1. BASIC HAND EXERCISE
2. SO WHAT?
3. L'ORIENTALE 1-6
4. THE BEAUTIFUL
5. THE APPLE
6. THE BALL
7. FLAT HAND KNIFE EXERCISE
8. DEFINING A BOX
9. THE MOVING BOX
10. THE GLOBE
11. POINTING THE FINGER
12. PLATE TURNING
13. OBJECTS, VARIATIONS, ETUDE

1. BASIC HAND EXERCISE

Exercise:

1. Stand in second position. Hands at waist level. Palm side up.
2. Make fists with both hands.
3. **Begin** with the **right** fist, **open** the fingers one by one to the count of five 1(thumb), 2 (index), 3 (middle), 4 (ring), and 5 (pinkie). **Close** the fingers starting with the sequence from the pinkie - 5 (pinkie), 4 (ring), 3 (middle), 2 (index), 1 (thumb)
4. Do this at least five times opening and closing the fingers back to the fist.
5. Now repeat the above sequence with the left hand.
6. Next, do both hands.
7. Extend arms forward in front of you and do both hands.
8. Extend arms above the head and do both hands.
9. Extend arms to side and do both hands.
10. Bring arms back to waist and do both hands.
11. Do wrist shaking upon completion of this cycle.

Benefits   Keeps the hands warm and flexible.
Enhances blood circulation.

2. SO WHAT?

Definition: This is the Basic Hand Exercise (1-2-3-4-5) done rapidly all at once as if to say "So What?"

Exercise:
1. Stand in first position. Breathe quietly.
2. Bend arms at the elbows. Maintain arms at waist level.
3. Do hand gesture forward, above the head and side-side.

4. Do each hand separately; then do both hands together.
5. Do hand gestures five times in each direction.

3. L'ORIENTALE (See Creative Body*Speak* Exercises Set 7.)

4. THE BEAUTIFUL

Exercise:
1. Stand in Artistic Zero.
2. Hold the thumb and index finger together in a circle.
3. Round, extend and separate the fingers. Hold the form.
4. Holding the form of "the beautiful," raise the right arm **up and forward** to shoulder level with the hand leading. Pause five seconds, then slowly lower the arm back down to the side.
   Repeat with the left arm.
5. Relax arms at side. Next, holding the form of "the beautiful," raise the right arm **up and out to the side** to shoulder level. Pause for five seconds, then slowly lower the arm back down to the side.
   Repeat with the left arm.
6. Holding the form of "the beautiful," raise the right arm **forward to up above the head**. Pause for five seconds, then slowly lower the arm back down to the side.
   Repeat with the left arm.
7. Holding the form of "the beautiful," raise the right arm **up and out diagonally**. Pause for five seconds, then slowly lower the arm back down to the side. Repeat with the left arm.
8. Holding the form of "the beautiful," **lower** the right arm **down and out diagonally**. Pause for five seconds, then slowly lower the arm back down to the side. Repeat with the left arm.
9. Do the movements in Step 4-8 with both hands. Do this pattern ten times.
10. Do the beautiful with the **windmill pattern** ten times.
    (See exercise above)

Benefits:
Increase dexterity of the fingers.
Release tension from the hands.
Learn to hold a form.

5. THE APPLE

Definition:
This is an exercise to perform before the ball exercise. It trains the hands to maintain form and increases dexterity of the wrists.

Exercise:
1. Stand in second position with knees relaxed.
2. Place an apple in your **right hand**.
3. Hold the left hand formed as a cup (fingers together) at waist level with the left arm extended.
4. Drop the apple into your **left hand**. Sense, feel and receive the weight of the apple. Keep the hand relaxed. Let the wrist drop naturally with the weight of the apple.

5. Repeat with the left hand giving the apple to the right hand, and the right hand receiving the apple.
6. The hands should go in a semicircle giving and receiving the apple.
7. Do the apple toss at least 25 times.

Benefits: Improve hand/eye coordination.
Engage the body in action and reaction.
Learn giving and receiving with the body.

6. THE BALL

Exercise:
1. Hold an imaginary ball in your **right hand**.
2. Throw the ball straight up in the air **at your side**. Follow the ball up and down with the eyes.
3. Receive and feel the weight of the ball. Let the wrist drop naturally when receiving the ball.
4. Toss the ball 10 times.
5. Repeat with the **left hand**.
6. Next, use both hands and toss the ball from right to left, then left to right in a semicircle.
7. Follow the ball with your eyes. Let the wrists drop naturally when catching the weight of the ball. Do this 10 times.
8. Next, while holding an imaginary ball in both the left and right hands, do the **windmill pattern**. (See above.)

The Benefits: Improve hand/eye coordination.
Sharpen the ability to focus and concentrate.

7. FLAT-HAND KNIFE EXERCISE

Exercise:
1. Place hands on a flat surface - wall or table.
2. Lift hands up in the air while maintaining the flat form and slowly walk back to the center of the room. Arms and hands should be at waist level.
3. Turn hands sharply so that palms face each other at waist level.
4. While maintaining the flat-hand knife form, sharply and swiftly extend the right hand and arm forward to full extension, shoulder level. The left hand and arm should follow immediately after the right.
5. Now both arms should be fully extended at shoulder level in front of the body. Palms should be facing each other while maintaining the flat hand form.
6. Both hands then simultaneously turn palm down and cut through the air like a knife with a quick crossing motion and then straight out to the sides at shoulder level.
7. Keeping arms at shoulder level and maintaining the flat-hand form, sharply turn hands palm forward one after the other.
8. Next, the hands slowly cut through the air and sweep down to the sides, one after the other, keeping palms forward. Hold.
9. Turn palms in to face the thighs one after the other.

10. **Repeat this sequence five times, beginning with #3.**

Benefit: Improve hand and arm coordination.

8. DEFINING A BOX

a. Small Box Exercise:

1. Stand in second position, with knees relaxed and bent.
2. Hold lower arms and hands at waist level with flat-hand knife form. Extend the hands forward. Palms inward. Keep the space between the two hands equal.
3. Beginning with the right hand and keeping the form, caress up the side of the box. Stop.
    Turn the palm sharply downward, caress the top of the box left to right and then back to the side edge of the box.
4. Turn the hand sharply with palm inward and caress back down the side of the box until in equal and neutral position with the other hand.
5. Repeat Step 3 & 4 with the left hand.
6. Next, beginning with the right hand and keeping the form , caress down the side of the box. Stop. Turn the palm up, and caress the bottom edge of the box from left to right and then back to the side edge of the box.
7. Turn the palm sharply inward and caress up the side of the box until in equal and neutral position with the other hand.
8. Repeat Step 6 &7 with the left hand.

b. Large Box Exercise:

Repeat the steps in the small box exercise, but just enlarge the space between the hands.

Benefit: Learn to form an invisible space; shape an invisible object.
Improve hand/eye coordination.
Makes mental images crisper and clearer.

9. THE MOVING BOX: Slow motion exercise, also called the *Moving Box Meditation*

Exercise: **Phase One**

1. Stand in first position.
2. Hold an imaginary box at waist level. Keep the form, and maintain the same distance between the hands.
3. Move the box to the right and return to center, keeping the box at waist level.
4. Move the box to the left and return to center, keeping the box at waist level.
5. Move the box up then down and return to center, keeping the box at waist level.
6. Maintain the shape with the same distance between the hands.

Phase Two

1. Stand in first position.
2. Place the right hand on the bottom of the box and move the box up, then place the right hand on the top of the box and move the box down and back to center.
3. Make sure the left hand keeps the form of the box as the right hand is moving the box up and down and back to center.
4. Switch and have the left hand move the box up and down at the same time that the right hand is maintaining the form.
5. The hands should be in neutral position. Now push the box side to side with hands take turns pushing and maintaining the form of the box.
6. Do up, down and side to side movements five times each.
7. Next, maintain the form of the box and circle right to left and then left to right. Do this phase five times each direction.

Benefit: Improve hand/eye and body coordination.
Calm the mind and the nerves.
Regulate heartbeat and breath.
Promote the inner flow of reflection.

10. THE GLOBE

Exercise: 1. Stand in second position.
2. Form a globe with your hands. Place left hand, palm side down at the top, and the right hand at the bottom holding the globe.
3. Keep the roundness of the globe. Turn the globe by bringing the left hand down at the same time the right hand is going up. Turn the globe in a circle at least 15-20 times. As you turn, make the globe smaller. Continue until the globe is as small as a tablet in the palm of your hand, then eat it.
4. Next, go from small to big.

Benefit: Improve hand/eye and body coordination.

11.   POINTING THE FINGER

Exercise: 1. Stand in second position.
2. Make a fist. Point with the index finger.
3. Start with **the right arm.**
4. Point to the right at shoulder level. Bring the arm back down to the side.
5. Point to the left at shoulder level. Bring the arm back down to the side.
6. Point up. Bring the arm back down to the side.
7. Point down. Bring the arm back down to the side.
8. Point diagonal up, bring the arm back down to the side.
9. Point diagonal down, bring the arm back down to the side.
10. Repeat with **the left arm**. Do this exercise 10 times with each arm.
11. Then movements 4-9 with **both arms** 10 times.
12. Next, do pointing the finger with the **windmill pattern.**

Benefit: Improve hand/eye and body coordination.

12. PLATE TURNING

Exercise: 1. Go to a flat surface - wall or table. Place hands on the object.
Lift hands up in the air and while maintaining the flat form, slowly walk back to the center of the room.
2. Turn the hands over. Imagine you are holding a plate in each hand. Keep fingers together.
3. Make a slow spiral turn **inward** toward the body with the **right** hand. Continue to spiral until you have made a complete circle. Do the same with the **left** hand. Do not lose the form of the hand.
4. Do five slow spiral turns with each hand, then, do ten spiral turns with both hands.
5. Next, do spiral turns **outward** with each hand five times, and then, with both hands together ten times.
6. Practice with a real plate and a paper plate to get the feel of the weight of a plate.

Note: **Make sure you don't spill the contents that are on the plate!**

Benefit: Adapt the whole body to the movement of the hand with the plate.

13. SUBJECTIVITY, OBJECTIVITY and beyond

Description: We live with objects every day. They vary in shape, size, color, texture, weight, strength, and usefulness. How aware are we of how we touch, see and use objects? How do we handle and manipulate the object? Is it real or imaginary, visible or invisible? Animate or inanimate? Do we have conscious awareness and an appreciation of the objects we are using?

Below is a table describing subjective and objective use of the object:

Mime Subjective	Mime Objective
Person	Object
Performer	Performed
Maker of illusion	Illusion of the object
Minimum movement	Maximum movement
Stillness	Motion
Being	Doing
Interior	Exterior
Me	It

Attention on the Object:

When we "talk about" the object itself, we give dry information, tell the story, and relay the facts. Describing the object is scientific. The object just is. We use it and witness what we do with it or what happens to it.

Attention on the Subject:

When we "move with the object," we should become it, be with it. Color, emotions and gestures of the personality can animate and add sparks when working with the object.

Exercises: Being with an Object:

1. Pick any object.
2. Feel and sense the texture and weight of the object.
3. Carry the object. Be aware of the weight and how your body moves with the object. Be with the object 100%.
4. Follow the contours and lines of the object.
5. Breathe with the object.
6. Imagine you and the object, are one.
7. Be aware of hand & eye coordination.
8. Work one object at a time.

Suggested objects

1. Ball
2. box
3. apple
4. lampshade
5. book
6. vase
7. bottle of wine
8. candle holder
9. hat, scarf
10. place mat
11. pillow
12. leaf
13. feather
14. wooden stick

Object Shape Shifting:

Toss or exchange one object and receive another. Improvise! You can do this alone or with a partner. Play with the object and know it kinesthetically before you toss it and, then, after you catch it!

Example

Pass an object, an **apple**, your partner receives a **cane**.
Pass a **hat**, your partner receives a **banana**
Pass a **pen** your partner receives a **sword,** etc.

Defining an Object:

Find objects in sets of three, which characterize "**smaller than me, as big as me, bigger than me.**" Try to work with each object, and then develop.

Examples:

A **stone** is **smaller than me**. A **boulder** is **as big as me**.
A **mountain** is **bigger than me.**

Thread/String/Rope
Kleenex/Towel/Curtain
Match/Torch/She sun
Twig/Branch/Tree/forest
Box/Window/Door

Benefits: Develops and sensitizes one to the art of touching.
Develops the sense of observation.
Increases eye/hand coordination.
Improves dexterity.
Allows you to discover more about your self.
Result in mental/physical balance.
Helps you to respect and use your hands when you need them.
Helps you begin to identify more with objects in the environment.
Develops and sensitizes one to the art of touching.

Note: Develop your dexterity with various other objects to train your hands to handle any object as faithfully as possible.

Creative Body*Speak*™ Exercise Set 9

ARM EXERCISES
    1. **WRIST SHAKING**
    2. **WINDMILL PATTERN**

1. WRIST SHAKING

Exercise:

1. Hold hands and arms above the head.
2. Shake the entire arms by activating the movement from the wrists.
3. Do this for 15-20 seconds.
4. Stop! HOLD the arms in willow tree position for approximately ten seconds, then slowly turn hands and wrists outward and sweep the arms down, caressing the spacing until arms are at side of body. Keep fingers together.

Benefits: Release tension. Improve circulation.

2. WINDMILL PATTERN Exercise:

1. Stand in first position. Relax arms at the sides. Look towards horizon. Breathe quietly.
2. Begin with the right arm. Lead up with the right wrist with right hand down. Bring the right arm up and forward to shoulder level. Stop.
3. Sharply turn the right wrist- right, at the same time the left wrist readies itself to come up and forward. Now at the same time, move the right arm to the right and sideways at the same time the left wrist is leading the left arm up and forward to shoulder level. Stop.
4. Sharply turn the left wrist - left, at the same time the right wrist gets ready to lead down with the hand up.
5. Sweep the left arm left and to the side at shoulder level at the same time the right arm sweeps down and returns to the side of the body. Stop.
6. Sharply turn left wrist with hand up. Sweep down with the left wrist at the same time the right wrist with right hand prepares to sweep up and forward. Left arm down and to the side while the right arm sweeps up and forward. Stop. This completes the cycle. **Do this cycle ten times.**

S T O R I E S

THE HORIZON *

As a child, I was fascinated with the horizon. I clearly remember my first encounter with this mysterious moving edge.

One day after school I found myself walking unconsciously in an unfamiliar direction. Suddenly I realized that I had gone far away into the fields. Looking to the horizon, with those majestic mountains of my birth place calling like a flute, I told myself: I should be home now, dinner will be waiting, my family is going to worry about me.

But under those blue skies the landscape captivated me entirely. I stood immobilized by awe. The thought formed: I want to go to the horizon, I want to live on the edge of the world, I want to *be* where the horizon is.

And my legs walked and walked and walked. The only focal point ahead of me was a single tree on the horizon line. One majestic tree. My fascination increased.

As I walked I decided: I'm going to meet this tree, it must be the tree of life itself. I had learned about the tree of life in school and now I was headed straight towards it. I could think no other thoughts. I could see only the tree.

The afternoon sun warmed me and I was not tired of walking. I just wanted to meet the horizon and rest under the tree. With the whole heart of a determined child I wanted to sit under that tree.

And then, I was looking up through its outstretched branches.

In the haze of my fatigue I concluded that this must be the edge of the world, surely. I had reached my destination. I sat down under the tree and read. And I understood, or pretended to understand, what I read.

Before I knew it the sun was going down and I had to get back home. I stood up and looked beyond the tree, and there, amazingly, was another horizon. I made a few attempts to walk toward it. I turned right, left, and found the horizon on all sides — calling me, embracing me.

As one sage said, "I wandered in pursuit of my own self. I was the traveler and I am the destination." In all of my travels since then I have walked toward that horizon and that tree.

---

* An autobiographical sketch. Unless otherwise noted, this and other pieces in this section have not previously been published.

THE DANCING EGG

Once, the family of Mr. Time and Mrs. Space gave birth to boy triplets. The one who was born first was called Yesterday. The next one born was called Today. And the last one born was called Tomorrow.

One day, many years later, they were walking in the forest together, Yesterday, Today, and Tomorrow, and they were having a discussion about the nature of existence: where did they come from, why were they here, where were they going, and so on ...

Suddenly, a bird flew from a tree and landed near them. To their amazement, she began to speak: "For the one among you who can answer this riddle, I will transform myself into a beautiful princess and live with him forever."

The riddle was: "How can an egg dance without breaking?"

Yesterday said, "I've seen worlds and time but I have no idea what you are talking about."

Tomorrow said, "I have no experience with such nonsense and *I* have no idea what you are talking about."

Today said, "I think I have an idea. There's one way an egg can dance without breaking and that's by being a mime."

So the bird transformed herself into a beautiful princess.

And then, she did something even more surprising. She reached into her pocket and took out an invisible egg. With a flourish, she cracked the egg into an invisible pan and proceeded to cook it over the invisible fire that she had prepared for the purpose.

When the egg was done, she offered some to Yesterday and Tomorrow. Then she took half of the cracked shell, transformed it into a crown, and placed it on Today's head, making him a prince. She placed the other half on her own head. Today smiled. They kissed a tender kiss.

And the clever princess took hold of Today's hand and away they danced — stopping now and then to pirouette, hand-in-hand — together.

THE MOUSE AND THE WORD

There was a mouse who was hungry to Know. He didn't know exactly what, but he was determined. He thought the knowledge he sought must be high up on the shelf in the Big Book. So, he began to climb and was met by many obstacles.

At last, he reached the top. He was very excited. But the Big Book he found was jammed in between many other books and he was too little to move it.

To another, the situation might have been hopeless, but the mouse was clever and his teeth were sharp. Up to the top of the Big Book he climbed and began to eat. Soon he had eaten right down to the middle.

The owner of the Big Book began searching for a definition. He pulled the Big Book from the shelf but the word he was looking for was gone. He slammed the Big Book down on the arm of his chair, and the mouse, observing, almost jumped out of his skin at the noise.

The mouse smiled for he had found the Word and his stomach was full. It remained for him now to digest the Word in silence. And as for Man, he calls the whole situation a Mystery.

MADNESS & SANITY on BROADWAY

Encountering America's state of mind of the mid 60s

The event of 32 years ago that gave me the first clue or sign of what America was all about remains vivid in my mind today. It was a first encounter that prepared me for America's state of mind then as well as now. I came to understand through great effort the meaning of this event only after much struggle.

I Remembered few years earlier in Paris, watching the assassination of JFK on French television. With the astonishment of that momentary emotion I wondered, why would a great and rich country kill its president? I developed a keen sense of observation while living in America during the turbulent 60s.

I arrived in New York City via Montréal from Paris in June of 1964, as a visitor of my friends Moni & Mina Yakim, with whom I resided until I found my own apartment.

As an innocent immigrant, not yet knowing English, American history or culture, I just dived in. New York was a jungle of confusion for me. I focused on learning the language fast so I could catch up with my self-education and face the realities of my new adventure: the discovery of my America.

In 1965 I have my first American performance at the theatre of La Mama. etc. downtown in the neighborhood of Second Ave. I offered classes in different schools, spoke enough English to get by, and read a lot.

Some of my performances depicted in silence and movement those personal observations, made through the artist's eyes. These were my own efforts to "understand" the western culture in which I chose to learn and develop my artistic career.

Then one day a street encounter gave me a real clue of the diseased symptoms and the way of thinking of America in its un-united "state".

I was walking on Broadway between 82nd and 84th streets, happy but contemplative about the strangeness of being here. I considered myself to be a physically, mentally, fit and healthy individual, and I was simply glad to be in this country.

I met a friend, actually an acquaintance whom I had known some time ago, and as we greeted each other, I asked him where he was going. He said, "I am going to see my psychiatrist." I thought to myself that to see a psychiatrist one must be mentally unbalanced or unable to cope with reality. So, I said with honesty, "Is something wrong? he then reacted very defensively, "No." he shouted, "If you don't have a psychiatrist then something is wrong with **you**," he said and disappeared into the crowd.

I was transfixed, planted firm on the ground, as dumbfounded as if I had just been struck by lightning on that beautiful and sunny day. My mind went blank. Shocked to the core, I thought about the irrationality of this person's behavior, his twisted logic, and his distorted perception of reality.

I couldn't understand then, that such a mentally disturbed individual, jump to a false conclusion about me and dare to judge me as abnormal because I did not have a psychiatrist. I found it to be utterly outrageous and insulting to my intelligence.

My thoughts raced for a conclusion or resolution as I woke up out of my stupor. Smiling to myself, I processed and absorbed this event. I identified and analyzed what had just occurred with my natural sense of objectivity, in order to make sense of it without being mentally injured by the distortion I had just witnessed. I found myself greatly amused with a deeper smile.

I realized and told myself, "my dear Samuel, you have just witnessed a glimpse of insanity and twisted reality. Now, you know that your have come to an immense insane asylum. This asylum is caught in a trap of false identities, distorted realities that have become a norm that relies on psychiatrists and external authorities, using them as an escape form facing the truth as it is."

This innocent nouveau immigrant suddenly understood the scope of his survival: that one has to be mentally strong and healthy to face the irrationalities of the majority - irrationalities which are considered a norm in this society.

I developed a safety valve called

"KEEP ME SANE IN THE MIDST OF MADNESS."

This valve of thinking objectively with common sense kept the flame of sanity alive in me, in spite of the imbalances that I had to deal with. I sharpened more my intellect to carry my artistic work creatively.

I developed a keen sense of observation, an ability to identify irrationalities and reject them in order to keep my sanity alive. I used my objectivity to stay logical and practice honesty in spite of the popular belief that it does not pay.

I identified reality as it was in regard to my emotions, the cheating and lying that were commonplace, and the "mystical" ideas that create problems where none exist. My experiences and involvement in my newly adopted and discovered country, made it possible for me to practice freedom of thought and action.
So my motto was and is to actively say to myself

"KEEP ME SANE IN THE MIDST OF MADNESS."

to stay alert and consciously awake to any winds of change, and be armed with a healthy sense of life and determination to be creatively happy, and above all, increasing kindness to all.

That event — an immigrant's encounter with madness and sanity on Broadway, New York City of 1965, gave me a shining glimpse of what was going to be my American Experience and a great lesson in my life.

From Le Centre du Silence Newsletter *"The MovingEdge"* Vol. 1. No.1. Fall 1991
Copyright © 1991 Samuel Avital

THE BEGINNING AGAIN*

Once upon a time, after a great cataclysm that almost obliterated life on this planet, a small group of peasants, who were very old, were the only survivors of the global disaster. They were struggling to survive by farming the blighted earth. But the earth was so damaged that their efforts to cultivate a few food crops were in vain.

Finally, in desperation, one aged man, wiser and more courageous than the rest, proposed to go out into the world in search of food. The other villagers were too frightened, discouraged, and weakened by illness and hunger to accompany him, so he decided to set out alone.

He found a path into the large dark forest that stood on the edge of the village fields. As he entered the forest's shadowy depths, he began to feel uneasy, and with good cause. No sooner had he reached a point where he could no longer see the village fields behind him, than a host of strange and fearsome creatures began to attack him. An upright writhing serpent crept up behind him, a hairy crawling beast without a name threatened his ankles, a sharp-taloned flying thing with great flapping wings descended from the sky upon him.

Despite his terror and infirmities, for he was very old, the man fended off the terrifying apparitions as best he could, knowing he had to continue on his quest for food.

Suddenly he heard a sound like none he had ever heard before — a haunting wail of utter misery, the thin and pitiful cry of an abandoned child. He could not possibly ignore it. He stepped off the path and made his way through the trees and underbrush, following the reedy cry as if entranced.

Pushing aside a leafy branch, he stepped into a small clearing. He saw before him the ruins of an ancient temple, its stone walls covered with moss, its cracked columns grown round with vines. The cries seemed to come from within the temple, so he mounted the worn stone steps and entered through a low, arched doorway.

Once his eyes had adjusted to the dim light inside, he saw a small figure huddled in front of a simple altar. It was moaning softly, rocking back and forth, its head bent upon its knees and half hidden by its encircling arms. He crossed the uneven marble floor and knelt in front of the strange little being. Reaching out a weathered hand, he lifted its head so that he could look at its face.

But what was this? The being had no face; its head was featureless, a smooth white oval, without eye or mouth or nose or ear, as blank and seamless as an egg.

He drew back, horrified, staring at this human form that looked sightlessly towards him for a moment and then quickly covered its terrible blank face with its hands, as if anguished by the revelation of its deformity.

The old man remained motionless, battling his impulse to flee from this travesty of humankind. Frightened and bewildered as he was, he sensed that the creature was suffering almost beyond belief. Tears came to his eyes and he felt his heart expand. Instinctively he reached out to the poor miserable creature and embraced it. It collapsed against him, its shoulders shaking with sobs.

Steeling himself against the horror of that blank visage, he cradled its head gently in his hands and turned it up towards him. Gazing intently at its eyeless face, as if to will a response into existence, he caressed the featureless oval. Its skin was soft and flawless, like that of a baby.

He felt an odd sensation growing in his hands. They were warm, so warm that they tingled. They seemed to move without his willing them to do so. Quickly they began to mold the little creature's smooth resilient flesh, making an indentation for eyes, shaping a nose, a mouth, ears. His hands moved now more rapidly and deftly until a fully human face, which seemed to have been waiting for a touch such as his to take form, looked back at him.

For a long moment, he and the newborn person gazed into each other's eyes. And then the person, whose fresh and perfect features reminded him of everyone who had ever been dear to him in the past and who might become so in the future, smiled. With this benevolent and grateful smile, which the old man matched with a joyous smile of his own, the two joined hands and walked out together into the waiting world.

A FISH STORY *

Once, there was a fish who lived in the great ocean, and because the water was transparent, and always conveniently out of the way of his nose when he moved along, he didn't know he was in the ocean.

Well, one day the fish did a very dangerous thing for a fish. He began to think: "Surely I am a most remarkable being, since I can move around like this in the middle of empty space."

Then the fish became confused because of thinking about moving and swimming, and he suddenly had an anxiety paroxysm, and thought that he had forgotten how. At that moment he looked down and saw the yawning chasm of the ocean depths, and he was terrified that he would drop.

Then he thought: "If I could catch hold of my tail in my mouth, I could hold myself up." And so he curled himself up and snapped at his tail. Unfortunately, his spine wasn't quite supple enough, so he missed.

As he went on trying to catch hold of his tail, the yawning black abyss below became ever more terrible, and he was brought to the edge of a total nervous breakdown.

The fish was about to give up, when the ocean, which had been watching with mixed feelings of pity and amusement, said, "What are you doing?"

"Oh," said the fish, "I'm terrified of falling into the deep dark abyss, and I'm trying to catch hold of my tail in my mouth to hold myself up." So the ocean said, "Well, you've been trying that for a long time now, and you still haven't fallen down. How come?"

"Oh, of course, I haven't fallen down yet," said the fish, "Because, because — I'm swimming!"

"Well," came the reply, "I am the Great Ocean, in which you live and move and are able to be a fish, and I have given all of myself to you in which to swim, and I support you all the time you swim. But here you, instead of exploring the length, breadth, depth, and height of my expanse, are wasting your time pursuing your own end."

From then on, the fish put his own end behind him (where it belonged) and set out to explore the Great Ocean.

---

* A new rendering of an ancient tale told to Samuel by his grandfather. Previously published in *MimeWorkbook* (Wilmot, WI: Lotus Light Publications, 1982-85).

* The "Beginning" Story was developed in the early seventies to illustrate dramatic elements for the students of the Mask Workshop's last class application performance. This story is still used as a final application for all *BodySpeak*™ workshops.

THE GAZELLE OF THE DAWN

Near a tree, in a green valley,
Beside a blooming hill.
Now — before the sun — on the horizon,
A silhouette appears:
A gazelle with bright eyes
Like the sun rising.

The sun's rays pass through the gazelle to me.

She approaches with her gentle walk
And stops just there,
Facing me with clear and steady eyes.
She has been grazing on flowers.
In her mouth is a flower.
She bends and places it in my lap.

I sit in total stillness.

Then, she walks back her way
To the horizon.
And as she walks,
My eyes do not leave her steps.
I count seven times that she stands in the field
And turns her head to look at me again.

The seventh time, at the top of the hill,

On that infinite line of the horizon.

PENSÉES and REFLECTIONS

Samuel's Teaching Words

Nothingness

Children are "nothing." When they fall, they are "nothing." If you are "nothing," you don't have the consciousness of tension, you are relaxed and you don't resist gravity, you cooperate with it. Only when you realize this "nothingness" can you do something.

Wisdom

Wisdom is knowledge properly applied to the affairs of the world; it is spiritual passion. King Solomon knew this, but few rulers of men have followed his example.

Spontaneity and Wisdom

It is possible to have a marriage, a unity, between the wisdom that comes from the experience of many difficult and painful lessons and the spontaneity and passion of youth, but it is very rare. Youth is busy with passion. The excitement of the wise man is larger than the excitement of youth.

Enlarge your idea of spontaneity. Spontaneity can be directed. So can passion, especially by the artist.

Teacher/Trickster

True teachers not only live the truth, they love the truth they live. But in fact, that truth, for the students, is a lie until they investigate it for themselves. So the teacher plays out his or her own role — being simple, stupid, outrageous, a trickster, whatever, luring the students on, sometimes satisfying their expectations, sometimes frustrating them, always testing, measuring, so that the students will measure their own something-ness. Even false teachers, with their half truths, can unwittingly aid in the quest if the students learn to relax and not force the issue, if they learn that in all their struggles what they are looking for is already looking for them.

Student-Teacher-Mentor Relationship

Both teacher and student know; one remembers, and one has forgotten. When they get together, they remind one another.

Give and Take

A teacher is one who takes what he or she is given and gives what cannot be taken.

From "Advice to a Young Mime"* for a young artist

So, my dear friend, you have decided to explore this marvelous art of mime — a territory unknown to many — and presumably your decision is motivated by sincerity and the honesty of your being.

If your motives are profound enough, that is, if they are not limited by time and space, this path will be full of great surprises and will unveil before you that which is considered the "invisible world" beyond. With this in mind let us see if you are well equipped with guidelines to lead you to success — to know yourself.

The art of mime, magical in many ways, is the ultimate language of silence, a universal language in itself that will give you access to the most hidden places of your being, places where you are one with all creation. It is, my friend, an adventure that will fulfill you totally — when the time is ripe, and as long as your honesty and sincerity remain unfettered.

As an adventurer, you must know that the path drawn on the map is not the same as the real path. The map is only an indicator of where to go, only an instrument to lead you onward.

The instrument with which you play this art-venture is your own body and, as an instrument, it has to be tuned. It is the house in which you live, breathe, and move.
 * From the French article "Experience d'un Jeune Mime" by Samuel. This article was translated for this publication as "Experience of a Young Mime."

On Being an Artist

In the evolution of civilization, the essence of the human being has been hidden from immediate awareness. This basic fact has caused an attribution of the artistic sense to visions of "other worlds," when in truth the reality of every human being is Artist.

Mime and Dream Making

I will give you my own definition of mime, as I see it after thirty years of practice. For me it becomes a multidimensional reality that transcends the communication with words that are attached to the only sense dimension that we have.

That other dimension, from my experience, is compared somehow to the dream world. You cannot write with words — you can, but in 500,000 volumes — you cannot write the dream. The dream has signals and symbols that communicate. Mime can help to work that dimension of dreams here — in the waking state. In other words, once the tool is sharpened enough or realized enough, the mime will fantasize, will write, will sculpt this fantasy in space. And that is an act which we call, in English, to perform.

Since I am a cutter of words, I am going to cut this word also and say Per/form — PER/form — per - per - per - purr - purr — the cat purr — purr —per form PRE form — in other words, you work your ideas in a certain way and PRE - Form them."

The Mask

A mask can mean many things. It may be thought of as a vessel that holds light, the vibration of dots captured in matter, the appearance connected with the essence, a tool for the creation of specific dramatic effects, an automatic depository for aspects of ourselves we don't understand, an edge, an onion layer. Every time you take off one mask, there is another.

A mask is a tool for communicating. It veils or unveils. A mask is a channel, an avenue, a threshold, for allowing expression to flow and to come out from within.

Verbal Abuse

We live in a new Babylon — an entangled web where the great danger lies in the inability to communicate simply. Complicated terminologies present great obstacles to communication; the words are not meaningful enough to convey the ideas in simple terms. It seems we are in love with useless complexities.

The Three Gates

There is a proverb which says that every word should pass through three gates before being uttered. At the first gate the gatekeeper asks, "Is it true?" At the second he ask, "Is it necessary?" At the third he asks, "Is it kind?"

Life-Long Laughter

Laughter is the high road to long life and self-healing. Laughter lightens us. We call the effect levity. Laughter elasticizes us. It keeps us supple. It releases our tensions. If we are laughing beings, we prolong our lives. We are concerned here not simply with life extension — why prolong mediocrity or misery — but with life expansion, from within. When we laugh, the whole system vibrates: the diaphragm dances when we laugh; the cells themselves dance. If we don't furnish our cells with this dancing vibration, which we call "laughing," we are robbing them of life. Laughter is a potent transformer.

Mentally Dead, Biologically merely existing

It is sad to observe these days that most of humans on this planet, pretend to be free while actually they are in a self-imposed prison, mentally dead, and biologically existing, merely living. This sad observation increases my motivation to give those who are ready to receive the tools and think more of themselves.

ANECDOTES and BON MOTS

Collected from Samuel's books, notes and other writings,
public lectures, workshops, seminars
and private conversations.

THE WORD BANK ECONOMY

My grandfather once told me that when we are born we were given a certain number of words in our **'word bank.'** If one uses too many words (like over spending too much) it empties our word bank account, they become overdrawn, or we become mute. So, when we use words only when necessary we practice word economy.

My grandfather's words made a very great impression on me as a young boy, no doubt contributing to my decision to make my life work in the Theater of Silence.

Words are only one of the ways to communicate; 99% of our real communication, however, occurs in silence, through your body language.

I highly recommend to practice one day of silence a week to achieve the ability to **speak less and do more** and **produce more and consume less** — practicing consistently the practical wisdom of the **word economy.**

First class in Boulder, Colorado,1972

I AM NOT A HUMAN BEING , I AM A HUMAN BECOMING:
THE IMPORTANCE OF BEING AN INDIVIDUAL

My friends, let me tell you one great truth today. The most important and essential value in the universe is the individual human being, capable of creative genius to manifest events, invent most unexpected values to benefit humanity.

The future belongs to the individual, the artist, the creator of new way of thinking—the individual who is a leader, who dares to think, to create, and has a fearless attitude to shape the future with utter simplicity, one who ignores the ways of the herd, and dares to be unique with humility and happiness.

All these characteristics have been and will always be in the healthy sense of being the creative artist. Most artists aspire to these values, to shape the un-shapeable and dare to say the unsaid with color, movement and sound. The future is shaped by such beings who soar while others crawl.

Strive to develop these characteristics and you will be most happy being alive and well, and always ready and generous enough to help others see the sun, the light of the one who dares to look within, and express without fear the murmurs of the heart, the élan of balance.

I declare the permanent state of happy existence to you by saying that,
I am not a Human Being — I am a Human Becoming.

On Self-Leadership, and the Importance of Individual Independence, 1972

HEAR, SEE, DO and UNDERSTAND

When I hear, I forget. When I see, I remember. When I do, I understand.   So, if you really want to learn and know how to HEAR, to SEE, to DO, and to ACT, you must make the effort to be present 100% all the time. Knowledge without proper and related action is utterly worthless. Wouldn't you agree?.

Demonstrating principles of body honesty to the International Summer Mime Workspace of 82

WHO IS LEADING YOUR LIFE?

Who Is Writing Your Script? Be The Author And Play the Lead Actor In Your Life, NOW. Use and explore the proven techniques of **Body*Speak*™** exercises to Unleash The Fearless Creative Power Within You.

In a public lecture/workshop 1991

"IN THE BEGINING WAS THE WORD"
BEFORE THE WORD, THERE WAS MOVEMENT.

Movement is vibration, life, vision, the stuff of creation and the essence of everything. An intelligent being thinks and talks, an emotional being sings, a totally integrated conscious being thinks, talks, sings and moves…ACT!

In a public park lecture/workshop 1978

REMEMBER and REALIZE for SELF-GUIDANCE

Identify and eliminate laziness and dishonesty in yourself and around you, Live passionately without guilt. Be always ready, alert, creative and responsive to the beautiful and vibrant life within you.

Happiness is your natural state of being and does not depend on anyone else but your own self. Enjoy 100% every present moment of your life . Remember! Your life is your only moment in eternity, precious and full with joie-de-vivre, a potent point of power. Give more than you take.

Focus your energy with vitality to produce values and earn your super happiness — your natural state of being. Happy Days Are Here - Great Days Are Coming. "Vive La Vie, Vive L'Amour, Vive La Liberté, Vive La Difference."

In a public lecture on honesty and laziness, Boulder, Colorado, Nov. 3, 1990

SEIZE THE DAY, SHAPE THE SPACE

When you practice the Presence Zone exercise you seize the moment, what I call elasticizing time and space you will learn to be and become a lion and rule your kingdom, learn to be like an eagle, soar above the crowd and be truly free, or be a sheep, follow the crowd and get slaughtered. That is the sane conscious choice for one to make to live totally. There are no excuses.

On Masks and Sticks, 1972

WHAT IS A GENUINE BEING ?

Not every guitar-scratcher is a musician, Not every white face in town square is a mime or clown, Not every house painter is a Picasso, Not every menu writer is a poet.

In a public park lecture/workshop, 1978

IN BRIEF

Samuel's
Small Words for Big Things

Make New Mistakes
Mistakes are useful, for we all can learn from them.
After you are **perfect**, then you make mistakes again, so why wait?
Enjoy your mistakes, and master the way to correct them.
Please, I am just asking you to always be sure to **make NEW mistakes**,
now that you know how to correct them creatively.

How to stop living in constant conflict with yourself
Most people live in a conflict with themselves by saying one thing and doing another. The thought and the action are contradictory, consciously and unconsciously—
this separation between mind and body.
The only remedy to this disease is to train yourself to **do what you say you will do, and say only what you really intend to do. T**his way you will align your thought and action and eliminate the conflict. You are not a split person who says one thing with the mouth and another with the heart. We call that human trait integrity.
This is the secret of being complete within yourself.

A Genuine Artist
Three ways to recognize the genuine artist:
lucidity, urgency, and impeccability.

Courage
Courage is a cloak you wear again and again
until every cell in your body is named, *Courage.*

Youth, Age ?
Youth is not an age — it is a fluidity of being.

The Art Of Mime Is The Art Of Life
The process of learning and mastering the art of mime, or the art of life,
is the 'suppling' of the spine — the real spine, or the spine of understanding.
Your body will respond readily to the expressions you wish to act out,
on the stage or in life. When you have a supple spine you really can feel
the power of the freedom of movement.
The point in this spine work, is to become aware of your whole body structure,
your skeleton — what supports your frame and bone structure,
your 'beginning' and your 'end.' Think about that.

Self = Etzem = Power
The word for "**self**" in Hebrew is the root word for "**bone**" ("etzem" which also means "**power**"). Inside the bone is the marrow, what makes us be physically alive. So when I say "**I am**" or "**myself**" I am aware
I am referring to my bones,
the frame of my existence now, my immediacy of being.
So, you can understand that the root of our being here is this bone structure
we are trying to learn about in this session. Did I give you enough hints
about the importance of you and I being here now?

Separate In Order To Unite
We separate and work each part of the body,
isolating and breaking down the whole
into small movements (atoms),
so later we can put them all together,
back to their wholeness and fullness of self expression.

Your Bones Will Remember
What is learned must be applied immediately.
What is learned with the body is never forgotten.
Your bones will remember. Be assured of that.

There Is No Vacation
Once you have chosen a path, a direction, a project, a mission,
remember, there is no vacation, nothing to vacate.

Push and Pull = Expansion and Contraction
Relaxation is a push and pull of the muscles at the same time,
an expansion and a contraction process,
which is happening each moment of our life's activities.
When you become aware of this law and apply it, your everyday life
becomes impeccably balanced and harmonious with remarkable ease.

Teach What You Want To Learn
When you show or teach someone something
you have not yet mastered and embodied,
you are killing them.
Ponder that!

Eye Control
The development of the person is told by the control of the eyes.

You Are An Open Book
Even the smallest movements you make reveal yourself.
There are people who can READ body movements.
Most of our communication happens with movement and silence,
as we have demonstrated in this workshop.
You know that!
So, my friend, you are an open book, for those who know,
and a closed book for those who don't know.
Therefore you are known and unknown at the same time.
Do you get it?
By simply knowing this fact, you can make your life.
Become a more human and more creative artist
in everything you do.

The Space Between
Be aware of the space between thought and action.
Music happens in the spaces between the piano keys.
The great actors use the silence between words and movements.

Totally Here
Let the movement of the exercise remind you to feel that you are
totally here, not to project to another space, past or future.

The secret of the presence is a raised torso.

The Two Edges
When the two edges meet, there is a natural support.

The Center Support
Do not support yourself, allow the center of your body and
your movement to support you.

The Great Secret of The Universe!
We often forget and take for granted the everyday movement,
because we forget to breathe.
Remember! I asked you once in every session—
What is the great and the most obvious secret in the universe?
Make sure to always remember to breathe!

What is the "IT"
It is not just by words that energy is revealed.
It manifests everywhere, in every form or shape.
It exists, whether you or I am aware of it or not.
So please read and ponder again the "**Fish Story**."

The Edge of Limitation
Know your limitations and find the unlimited in them,
at the edge of limitation there you will find the unlimited.

A Beautiful Hand Is
If you try to form the hand, it becomes ugly.
If you leave it natural, it is beautiful.
Allow beauty to be.

Bread and Salt
On your table, bread, salt and wine should be present to teach you something.

Condensation
Everything in the world is a product of condensation.
When you observe this fact your wisdom will increase.

"This" Moment, "That" Moment
If the moment is constant, the future is assured.
When you are just aware of what you do,
the circumstances will be there in the near future.
Just do not interfere with the process,
let it happen after you invest your total attention
in this present moment.

Living Totally 100% in the Present
This mode of thinking and being means that whatever you do now
should be like the first time and the last time.
This increases the intensity of living totally in the present.

The Now Will Slap You in the Face
When you are fully and honestly present this very moment,
the Now will slap you in the face
with an increased amount of kindness.

The Circle of Movement
The leader and follower are a circle.
Every step you perform is a proof of this.
Without the first step there is no second step,
and before every step there was a first step.
So, which is the first and second step?
Ponder the circularity of motion when you walk.

Be A Self-Leader Not a Follower
When you don't need a teacher anymore, you have to drop him off a cliff or you won't grow and become
your own teacher. The idea here is for you to become your own self-leader, not a follower. Escape the
mass sheep consciousness we witness everyday. Self guidance is the best. You don't depend on me or
anyone else but yourself. That's called self-reliance. You have experienced this principle in this
workshop, and you see the aliveness of your body's responses working with you, for you. When I make
you aware of this fact — to become your own teacher, your own leader, I will consider that a success. I
am here to guide you until you become your own teacher. That is my purpose of being with you now.
Actually I am not a teacher.
I am here just to remind you of this fact you have forgotten. I repeat: become your own leader and
teacher. That is the purpose of this session of Leaders and Followers.

Time Edge
Just at the point when you are ready to quit, the work begins.
Are you ready to observe the nuance of this moment of quitting?

Eat When You Are Hungry
We must forgive ourselves and others very very quickly, if we want to survive.
Use this motto I live by that I learned from my grandfather:
**"I eat when I am hungry, I drink when I am thirsty,
and I forgive myself and others very quickly."**

The Happening of the Verb
If you verbalize about it, it doesn't happen totally.
It's when you do it that it happens.

You asked for It
You get what you need, what you deserve. You are the cause of all that
you make happen. Simply knowing and experiencing this fact will give
you a profound sense of freedom you never knew before.

"Unknown" Is Not Yet Known
"In the beginning was the word. Before the word there was motion,
vibration, movement — the source of all life."
The artist is the one who steps into the "unknown" and acts as though
it were just another day, that simple, eh!
Remember the "unknown" is some event that "is not yet known."
It has the potential to be known, if only you look for it,
because it is there and always looking for you.

"So What ?" Exercise
A concept and movement, a humorous and healthy response to anything that is overdone, or over chewed
or over talked, in order to keep your balance, a valve or a conscious ward against fanaticism or extreme
behavior, a remembering tool, a signal to keep the state of equanimity, an inner/outer balance in every
thought and action.

Little Movement
Every little movement has a line, a breath, a structure, and a center.

Self Control
Conquer your world, yourself, with quiet power and silence, in a relaxed way.

New Universe
Let the movement teach you how to breathe.
You will discover a whole new universe.

Words are not thoughts
Words are not thoughts; they are only one of the means to express thoughts verbally. Most of our ways of communication and expression of thoughts
are done with our bodies, with our movements.

Body Honesty, Word Honesty
You can twist the meaning of words and take them out of context, being dishonest,
but you cannot do this with the body, because you cannot turn your head 360 degrees without **discovering** your spine.   You do that by going to the edge of your limit of turning your head right or left without discovering **the pivot**. If you go beyond the limit of turning the head beyond the edge, you will discover the **pivot and the spine.**

This is what I call Body Honesty. You can lie with words but not with the body.
So, "mystery" is not to be searched and wondered about, "mystery" is to be lived.
It is in the body, in your bones, in your skeleton, in your structure. Get it?

The Doors are always OPEN
When a door bangs shut, most people are attracted to the noise
and get distracted by where all the attention is.
However, the time when the door is shut is the **exact moment**
when you should be looking for the next door that is actually open before you.
There is no need of "keys" but if you feel you need a "key" remember,
You are the key. Use it and enter the door.

Perfection
Perfect movement is not enough. It must be perfect spirit and intention, too.
The **intention to be perfect** and precise gives us **a sense of being perfect**.

Fearlessness
Living in a world plagued by the disease of violence, the only logical cure
is to make a special effort to increase kindness toward oneself and others.
Functioning from this premise one become fearless and creative beyond imagination.

Three ways of learning

When my grandfather and I sat on a small smooth rock in his yard, after stamping the grapes rhythmically with my bare young feet, learning how to make wine, he told me that there are three basic ways of living and learning:

1. **The first** priority and purpose of life is **live to learn**, absorbing like a sponge, sharpening and using your intelligence to learn as much as you can, with increased curiosity.

2. **The second** priority and purpose of life is **living your learning,** mastering the practicality of your learning.

3. **The third** priority and purpose if life is to **tell a passionate story** of your experience, so others can also learn and benefit from your brief existence on this earth.

Over the years I reflected on this profound wisdom many times. I adapted these three processes of learning to most of my activities. (See the *"What is BodySpeak™?* article about the three phases of learning I use in my workshops and seminars).

From the first International Summer Mime Workspace, 1975, Boulder, Colorado

"Paradox"

Paradox is a deeply imposed conflict of intelligence
that is directed only to one small aspect of being.
In reality this is a tool in the hands of people
who manipulate others to their own benefit.
Go ponder on this and you will find whatever you will find.

Talking about "Conscious Innocence" in class, 1975
(See **"Defintuitions"** for more on Conscious Innocence)

Silence

Silence, the 'Golden Bit,' is the fence of wisdom.
When you *know*, you bite the Golden Bit.

An anonymous French proverb I love to remember says:
"Si ce que tu vas dire n'est pas plus beau que le silence ne le dis pas."
"If what you are going to say is not more beautiful than silence do not say it."

DEFINTUITIONS

**A few terms, words, expressions linked to specific movement experiences
during the workshops over the years.**

Application   An occasion to concretize learning.

Artistic Zero   Natural posture. Physically a perfect vertical line. Focused and totally present mentally and spiritually in all living situations. The state of being 100% totally in the present moment

Basketology of Silence   Weaving a fabric of silent communication (achieved during the "Eye-Knot" exercise); an awareness that space is not empty but has texture that can be woven to create meaning.

Bewilderness   A place or state of unrefined energy where one lives in confusion, or potentially — fusion.

Le Centre du Silence   A neutral space/time in absolute silence and stillness from which clarity of sight can be manifested on all planes with an amazing simplicity. The **Centre of Silence** is an invisible dot in an infinite circle, it is a good place/time to function from in total calm and poise in any situation you are in. Teach yourself to always respond to life from a **center of silence**.

Conscious Innocence   A living state and a natural quality of being, where one feels, becomes and is totally with the child innocence and consciously knows it. Paradox? Well, when one knows with certainty that paradox does not exist, then this state of conscious innocence is totally understood and lived.

Clowns, genuine artists, musicians, painters, writers, actors, and yes, mimes, also have this beautiful quality of being, which is a great source of true and potent creativity, a kind of innocence, but aware. Einstein and some other scientists had it. It is known that the gaze of a consciously innocent being is the most powerful in the world. It can be, what people call a "**miraculous**" event.

If you did not lose your innocence after childhood, you will begin to know it and understand it from the depth of your being.

Cosmic Accordion   The journey between the infinitely small and the infinitely big, back and forth and back again.

Dancing Diaphragm   An action that occurs during laughter as tension is released, a state of relaxation where learning occurs.

Elasticizing The Present	Stretching the moment, elongating the moment; being 100% present; breathing the Great Breath.
Elephant-in-the-Dark Mentality	Seeing only the part, not the whole.
From Ecstasy To Lunch	The ability to return to zero from any state at any moment.
Grasping The Void	Working in the space between thought and action, between the yes and no. **The music happens between the piano keys.**
Jump Into The Fire	Do that which you are afraid of, face your fears, dare to experience the edge, **envision yourself fearles**s.
Mental Mirror	The mirror of the mime; the screen of the closed eyelid on which you see yourself performing an action; **inner video.**
Minimum Movement, Maximum Expression	Small gestures can be the most meaningful. Dramatics serve their purpose but can be left at the stage door.
Natural Gentle Touch NGT	Used in the "snail" session; a guiding thought to sharpen awareness.
"Paradox"	"Paradox" is a deeply imposed conflict of intelligence that is directed only to one small aspect of being. In reality this is a tool in the hands of people who manipulate others to their own benefit. (See "Conscious Innocence.")
Performer, Performing, Performance are One	The one who is doing it, that which is being done, the state of being in it and watching it at the same time, all become as one whole reality.
Presence	Charisma is force of personality. Presence is the life force manifesting itself..
Relaxation	A conscious readiness to respond.
Responsibility	The ability to respond, creatively and immediately.
"So What ?" exercise	A concept and a movement, a humorous and healthy response to anything that is overdone, or over chewed or over talked in order to keep your balance, a valve or a conscious ward against fanaticism or extreme behavior, a remembering tool, a signal to keep the state of equanimity, an inner/outer balance in every thought and action.
"So What ?" Movement:	Bring both hands close to the abdomen, half closed and move them elegantly onward and upward while opening them with a dynamic surprise, and back. This exercise is learned fully with the **"Hands"** session

75/25 – for "this world"	25% of you is the observer. 75% is totally absorbed in what you are doing.
75/25 –for "that world"	25% of you is the BEING. 75% is totally the observer.
Worder/Worker	One who talks (words) **about** doing/one who does(work), moves and acts.

Samuel Avital

AFTERWORD

The Ultimate Object:
Overcoming Self-Created Obstacles
through Mime

By Jane Evenson

Gravitational Tango

Birth is the original experience of disorientation. The world presents itself as a three-dimensional obstacle course that we must learn to navigate. In the first year of life the child embarks on a hero's journey to attain the vertical dimension and walk upright. But as consciousness develops, physical obstacles presented in exterior space become pebbles in the road compared to imagined obstacles created in interior space. These self-created obstacles are a greater impediment to physical navigation than we might realize, as participants in Samuel Avital's Body*Speak*™ workshops soon discover.

Call it *gravitational tango*—a dance of self and other in three-dimensional space. It's the theme of a wonderful film in which a blind man drives a Ferrari and teaches a young woman to dance but nearly crashes against deeper self-created obstacles: "When you get tangled up in life, tango on."

Avital's work refines at the deepest levels the ability to navigate life through all its perplexing entanglements—physical, emotional, mental, and spiritual. It is the very definition of "interactivity": a process whereby knowledge is embedded in bone, muscle, and sinew through action in a group-learning environment. Participation in a Body*Speak*™ workshop is an object lesson, quite literally, in the powers of kinesthetic learning and active imagination.

Developing "Stick Consciousness"

Take that simplest of objects: a stick. Because of its representational capabilities, Avital calls it "The Ultimate Object." Students come to the workshop equipped with a three-quarter-inch dowel about the length of a broomstick. It can become a magic wand, a sword, a scepter, spyglass, digging tool, fishing pole, broom, barbell, flag pole, walking staff, measuring rod, musical instrument, or most meaningfully in the workshop environment, a threshold. Avital uses a simple exercise to illustrate a principle.

"Take the stick in your two hands," he says. Then he illustrates the maneuver: "Hands shoulder width apart. Now lean down. The stick should be at the height of your ankles. Now step over the stick without letting go of it with your two hands. Simple."

Not so simple. No one can do it. Even after several attempts. The biomechanical tendency is to lift the stick while taking the step. The stick converts instantly from threshold to obstacle. "How to solve this problem?" Avital asks.

131

A few people start to get the knack of it, but with effort. They strain and groan, catching their feet, stepping on the sticks, dropping the sticks. Suddenly there is a cacophony of dropping sticks as frustration mounts. Then Avital explains the secret. Most people grip the stick too hard, hanging on for dear life. "Let's start over," he suggests. "We need to develop stick consciousness."

Try the workshop exercise yourself. A broomstick (without the broom head) will do, but a smooth dowel works best.

Step One

The first step is to learn to relax your grip. Cradle the stick in your hands—holding it loosely, hands shoulder width apart, palms open and up, fingers and thumb curved slightly inward towards each other to create a cylindrical space. Revolve the stick toward you with a quick, shaking motion—rolling it over and over in the hollow of your hands. This loosens the grip and stimulates the hands, increasing relaxation and alertness at the same time. Simple.

Step Two

The next step is to learn to measure your effort and the strength of your grip. Hold the stick vertically, grasping it lightly with your fingertips, resting it on the floor in front of the body midline, right hand close to the middle of the stick about six inches below the left, elbows relaxed and close to the body, eyes looking straight ahead toward the "horizon," not focused on the stick. With a staccato thrust of your right hand, propel the stick straight up through the hollow of your left hand and catch it with both hands close together near the end of the stick—without looking at the stick or letting it fly out of control. Release the stick to slide down through your hands again and catch it just before it strikes the floor.

Not so simple. But after a few trials a miracle happens. Through a subtle interplay of attention and relaxation, the body learns to measure distance, sets the grip at just the right strength and releases the stick with the proper measure of *élan,* a key word in the lexicon of Le Centre du Silence.

In Avital's definition, *élan* is the spirit of the movement, its energy signature and life force. It is like a spring or a trampoline bounce that recoils to gather force for the thrust. Low energy? Low spirits? Frustration? Fear? "Ah," says Avital. "That's part of the *élan,* the *tremplin* (trampoline) that you use to bounce back in order to propel yourself to greater heights."

Another key word in the Avital lexicon is the Kabbalistic term *kavanah.* As Aryeh Kaplan says, *kavanah* means many things: concentration, attention, devotion, intention, and more—"the sum being more than the parts." (Kaplan 1982, p. 118) Avital defines it as "the flame of attention"—the ability to be aware of the target, as in the Zen art of archery, without inhibiting the arrow's flight. Breathing helps, and a certain élan.

Step Three

Now that you have acquired "stick consciousness" in the vertical dimension, you are ready to master the horizontal. Hold the stick waist high in front of the body—elbows close to your waist, right hand palm up at the middle of the stick, cradling it loosely, index and middle finger of the left hand lightly touching the left end of the stick on the tip. Again, look toward the horizon, not at the stick.

With the élan you developed for the vertical thrust of the stick, now use the two fingers of your left hand to propel the stick sideways through the cylinder formed by the right hand. Again, catch the stick near the end, but this time just with the right hand. Be careful. Avoid pointing the stick toward fragile objects. It might be best to do this exercise outdoors. Repeat the process several times until you master the right-hand thrust-and-catch. Then reverse and try it several times to the left.

Step Four

The next step combines horizontal and vertical. Return to step one and resume rolling the stick. Now toss the stick up with both hands, letting go and reversing your hands, and catch the stick overhand at arm's length above your head. The ideal is to accomplish this maneuver without looking at the stick or above your head, focusing your gaze on the horizon throughout the move. At this point, though, Avital will say, "Be merciful with yourself." It is okay to look at the stick the first few times to avoid hitting yourself on the head.

After several visually aided successes, when you accomplish the catch without looking, the effect can be exhilarating. The uplift of the movement opens the chest and makes the heart beat faster. You have avoided danger. You fantasize momentarily about trying out for Cirque du Soleil. Avital contributes to the moment by signaling "Hup" as an acrobat would. You send the stick aloft again. Success is sweet. Now try the same maneuver, but catch the stick with one hand at a time, alternating left and right. You begin to feel like a warrior brandishing a spear.

Steps Five, Six, Seven...

In the workshop, the stick session lasts over an hour, with many variations of the exercises. Sticks are tossed back and forth among participants at various angles and elevations. Avital heightens the element of "danger" by sweeping the stick back and forth low across the floor, triggering whoops and a percussion of jumping feet. Again, there is a warrior-like release. The workshop has a shamanic feel. Children learn this way, spontaneously through mimicry. Adults have forgotten how.

Destination: Mastery

Now it is time to return to the threshold exercise and try it again. You are ready to practice a skill that in the art of mime is called "fixation"—the ability to fix one area of the body at a point in space and move the rest of the body around that point. It is of course easiest to use your foot as the pivot, because you can fix it in contact with the floor. But it is also possible to hold your head as a fixed point and move around that, or your shoulder, elbow, knee, virtually any part of the body.

In this case, you will "fix" the position of your hands. Remember: it was the tendency to lift the stick while stepping up that caused problems in the first place. Begin by holding the stick at the height of the ankles. Grasp it lightly with the fingertips. Focus on maintaining your hands at the level of an imaginary two-dimensional plane and pivot your body up and over that fixed level. Angle your hips slightly, if necessary. Breathe. Relax. Step over.

Now try the same maneuver at the level of the knees and then at the upper thighs. This requires good abdominal muscles and somewhat greater agility, but the same measure of *kavanah.*

If you followed the steps of these exercises and were not able to accomplish the maneuvers, do not lose heart. Verbal description is no substitute for the workshop and is only intended to provide the flavor of the experience. Avital gives a hilarious mime performance called "The Yoga Student" to illustrate the rigors of attempting to learn yoga asanas from a book: entangling and disentangling his limbs and repeatedly consulting the master *text* in an attempt to perfect the postures.

The Internal Map

On the path to developing "stick consciousness" workshop participants cross a number of thresholds. These are "ah-ha" moments where specific skills are embodied. The muscles begin to remember. An internal map develops. "It's like reaching for a pillow in the dark," says an ancient Chinese text, "throughout the body are hands and eyes." (Cleary 1977, p. 571, author's rendering of a slightly longer passage from the text translation) We feel our way, developing peripheral vision and the ability to scan and focus simultaneously as hunters and gatherers do: estimating distances precisely, anticipating obstacles, alert to the next move.

In *The Hand,* an intriguing study of the impact on human intelligence of the evolution of the hand, neurologist Frank R. Wilson quotes juggler Serge Percelly, who developed "an eye for tennis" and found his niche in life when he began juggling tennis rackets:

> Most tennis players look at the ball until it hits the racket, and I never did that. I could see exactly where the ball was going without fixing the ball. You have to do the same thing in juggling. You have to fix a point somewhere, *where you actually see a bit of everything*, (emphasis added) and that comes only with practice. You always know if it's a bad throw or a good throw when you do it, and you know if you're going to catch it or not. (Wilson 1998, p. 101)

The ability to "fix a point somewhere, where you actually see a bit of everything"—to scan and focus simultaneously —is a valuable skill. Tony Hiss calls this ability "to feel relaxed and alert at the same time" *simultaneous perception.* (Hiss 1990, p. 5 ff) It enables a hunter, or an actor, to "hit the mark." It is the juggler's *kavanah.* It helps a participant in Avital's workshop to step over the stick threshold with less effort. In the larger sense, it contributes to "perspective"—the capacity to take in the larger picture and consider other points of view while focusing on the issue at hand. Enlarged perspective contributes ultimately to wisdom.

Kinesthetic Intelligence

The ability to "know" if the toss of a stick is good is a kinesthetic skill. In simplest terms, *kinesthesia* is the sense of bodily presence and orientation in space we gain from the action of gravity on the vestibular system of the inner ear working in conjunction with proprioceptors in the muscles and joints and with support from visual, auditory, and tactile cues.

Howard Gardner, whose theory of multiple intelligences has been highly influential, includes "bodily-kinesthetic intelligence" on a list of seven "intelligences"—along with verbal-linguistic, logical-mathematical, musical, visual-spatial, interpersonal (self awareness) and intrapersonal (social skill). (Gardner 1995) Recently, he has added an eighth and ninth intelligence to the list: "naturalist intelligence," the ability of an individual to relate to nature, and "existential intelligence," the ability to think in terms of larger issues that might be termed religious or spiritual.

While it is true that individuals may be more or less adept in certain areas and in essence "specialize," Gardner acknowledges that types of intelligence are not discretely isolatable in practice. His chief contribution, a humane one, has been to elevate the value of abilities that have not held the privileged position accorded in Western culture to verbal-linguistic and logical-mathematical intelligence.

Yet some confusion can result from these distinctions, because multiple "intelligences" must work in conjunction to make possible even such familiar skills as hand/eye coordination. In fact, kinesthetic intelligence underpins all the other forms of intelligence Gardner distinguishes. The senses are so closely integrated in phenomena such as hand-eye coordination, we might as well refer to a "tacto-visual" kinesthetic sense. An excellent introduction to fundamental kinesthetic impacts on learning is provided by neurophysiologist and educator Carla Hannaford in *Smart Moves: Why Learning is Not All in Your Head*. (Hannaford 1995) By employing simple "Brain Gym" exercises originally developed by Paul Dennison, Hannaford achieved remarkable results working with children labeled emotionally or learning impaired.

In truth, bodily intelligence enhances all the ways we learn, including supposedly "head-centered" modes such as the verbal-linguistic and logical-mathematical. Verbal or musical skill depends upon a sense of rhythm, balance, and placement: "Proper words in proper places, make the true definition of style," said Jonathan Swift. Logical and mathematical ability also requires a sense of balance and proportion; mathematicians frequently describe the "elegance" of a proof. Spatial-orientational skills are kinesthetically based. Personal and social skills are anchored in the rhythms of the body: mental "balance" describes a state of health; people "in sync" communicate effortlessly.

The kinesthetic sense also plays a role in the development of subtler faculties: intuition, for example. In *Genius*, a biography of physicist Richard Feynman, James Gleick describes "physical intuition" as key to how some of the great minds work:

> Feynman said to Dyson, and Dyson agreed, that Einstein's great work had sprung from physical intuition and that when Einstein stopped creating it was because "he stopped thinking in concrete physical images and became a manipulator of equations." Intuition was not just visual, but auditory and kinesthetic.

When intensely focused, Feynman himself would roll about on the floor, murmur rhythmically, or drum his fingers. Gleick goes on to describe how "the process of scientific visualization is a process of putting oneself *in* nature: in an imagined beam of light, in a relativistic electron." He quotes science historian Gerald Holton: "there is a mutual mapping of the mind...and the laws of nature." (Gleick 1993, p. 244)

Chess players are also adept at internal mapping, which is why chess has long been used to teach rules of strategy to generals and business leaders. In a 1999 interview, Howard Gardner himself describes "a kind of meta-capacity," an ability "to step back and see the big picture and not be overwhelmed by the details of the moment." To accomplish this, he says, "some kind of space" opens up "in which you're able to conceive contingencies and events and, as in a chess game, project several steps ahead of where you are now." He wonders if this "meta-capacity" is a separate kind of intelligence, but notes that "it certainly is a rare kind of capacity," one he admits "we don't understand very well." (Kurtzman 1999, p. 97) The more familiar term for what Gardner struggles to describe, is not "meta-capacity" but "wisdom"—or at least a set of skills implicated in wisdom.

Gardner wonders about an intelligence beyond "expertise" that the musical conductor must have, which combines the "courage and finesse and charisma to get in front of a bunch of crusty old musicians and get them to behave and to perform at their peak." (Kurtzman 1999, p. 97) If a name is required for this capacity, it might as well be "conductor intelligence": an understanding of how things fit together and of what works—"conduct" in an expanded sense—combined with the ability to lead. Though not as lofty as "wisdom," this is clearly a skill that master teachers must possess, or enlightened executives.

What is really being described, though, is a high-order application of kinesthetic intelligence. A symphonic orchestration of bodymind competence: that embraces self-knowledge, knowledge of others and what motivates them, communication skill, powers of concentration and internal mapping, strategic sense and the capacity to make projections, and not least, a sense of rhythm or timing—knowing when, where, and how to do what for whom. It is also a kind of internal barometer; the reason why, when a decision is right, we say: "I just feel it in my bones."

The Great Puzzle

Let us look for a moment at another of the ways Samuel Avital teaches "bone-deep intelligence." He calls the exercise "The Great Puzzle." Workshop participants work in pairs. The object of the exercise is to get your partner to go from vertical to horizontal or vice versa by a series of maneuvers that you instigate with a gentle tapping motion Avital calls "The Snail Technique."

Think how a snail negotiates its way carefully across a surface: projecting its antennae to explore obstacles, then recoiling with a slight arch and gathering itself up for the next glide. The snail has its own élan. This is how you will signal your partner to move a part of the body—the shoulder or knee or elbow, for example—by tapping it gently as if with a snail's antennae and then arching the hand gracefully away. Your partner responds with a reciprocal movement, recoiling the shoulder gracefully away from you. The wisdom of the method is that it keeps the tapping from getting too rough. You apply an understanding of body dynamics and project a series of moves that will enable your partner to descend or ascend move-by-move without toppling over or getting impossibly contorted. The body becomes a puzzle you must solve.

The key to solving the puzzle is to consult your own "internal map" and feel what is possible while taking into account the limits of what your partner can do. The Great Puzzle becomes not only an exercise in strategy but empathy. It is also one of the many ways Avital teaches navigation of the internal map, a vivid illustration of how to overcome self-created obstacles, this time in partnership.

The workshop poses many such puzzles. To accomplish "The Eye-Knot," partners face each other and visualize a cord connecting their eyes. The object is to "tie" a knot in this cord without losing eye contact and breaking the cord. Mutual concentration becomes so intense that the participants do not notice Avital approaching with his imaginary scissors. Subversively, he "cuts" the cord and the startled puzzlers fall to the ground! The trick to performing The Eye-Knot successfully is to avoid too much analysis and let the body *think*.

Facing the Mask

Each orientational puzzle Avital poses is an exercise in kinesthetic strategy and another of many thresholds crossed in preparation for the culminating moment of the workshop: the mask session. In this final exercise—*moving* in more than one respect—the many elements taught in the workshop coalesce. A verbatim transcript of an actual mask session (portions of which are excerpted here) is provided in this *Manual* in the poetic essay, "Facing the Mask." Avital explains why the mask is used:

> When a person covers his face with a mask, he thinks his real face is hidden. He feels safe behind the facade, and he acts as though he were not seen. Faces customarily dominate expression. We are accustomed to watching faces; consequently, we rarely notice what emotions the rest of the body is expressing. There are muscles in the face that we tense even when we think we are relaxed. When the gesticulations of the face are concealed by some sort of covering, a mask, suddenly we take notice of the body. Then something startling is revealed. By covering the face, we discover the real face, the real self....

In the mask session, a capacity for "deep orientation" is revealed: the skill required to navigate subtle inner dimensions using the internal map. An inner guide emerges. Avital calls this guide "the presence."

The work with masks opens beautiful doors to us to be in touch with ourselves and to become aware of the presence, that formless guidance that springs up from the center of our being. This form of work opens new vistas of self exploration to the student.

With a partner, workshop participants prepare white masks of their own faces, called "neutral masks," using plaster gauze. Mask creation is a kind of meditative exercise in itself as you gently apply strips of gauze to your partner's face. "Take care," says Avital. "You hold your partner's life in your hands." The masks are allowed to dry and then carefully sanded, covered with coats of gesso and sanded again. By the final day of the workshop, the masks are smooth and ready.
At the beginning of the session, you are asked to sit on the floor to study your mask:

Observe the texture and other details. It's part of your skin that you have peeled. It's a replica of your physical face. Think no thoughts other than about the mask. Look at the shape of the features. Do not judge, just look. Look at the eyes. They appear as two holes that reach infinity. Become familiar with your face that you hold in your hands.

Then you put on the mask:

Take five million years to do this. No brusque movements. Every movement should be very conscious. With the mask on, keep the eyes closed. Breathe very calmly. Begin to feel your own facial structure under the mask. It is covered, as if by clothes.

You begin your journey:

Visualize yourself sitting in water up to your neck. It is the ocean. What you see is the horizon of the waters. Nourish the waters, the horizon, and ask who is behind the mask. It has no name. Is it your face?...Find the neutral one, the no-name one, the circle, the empty one within. That center of the circle is there living behind every being...

Now you begin to move:

Stand up using very slow motion. Who is behind the mask moving the body? It is a new physical being that you discover, but who is discovering it? Who is moving the body from the inside? The goal is to stand. Do not plan any movement. Let the one behind the mask move you.

Discover the inner guide:

Once you stand, get in touch with that presence...If we are aware of it, everything becomes fresh, as if for the first time. Let the presence walk, using the vehicle of the body. Any movement we do now is in the service of walking, with appreciation and reverence. The presence goes for a promenade. It is not limited in any way. Turn. When the head meets the limitation of the body, the presence continues. The presence will teach you to turn.

You play at shifting states and shapes and "see how the presence relates":

Be cold! Let coldness contract the body, as the presence stays remote, observing the expression of the body.... Now change; be hot! Immediately the body expands and droops, but the presence stays distant.

The body takes on archetypes. Be a warrior! The archetype of the warrior is one who knows his power and knows how to use it positively. Be a coward! Receive the universal coward in you.

Time drops away but for perhaps an hour you explore different environmental states, walking through water and sand and wind, conducting silent "dialogues" with other workshop participants. And then:

Come back to the original spot where you began. The presence sits like a king or queen. It knows how to sit. The one who is sitting has a right to be there. Turn the head to brush the horizon. Just the head. *C'est une noblesse de presence.* Close the windows and sit still in the waters. Very slowly, eyes closed, take off the mask and hold it facing you.

A realization dawns: the body itself is a threshold. We cross it every night in sleep and eventually in death. We can learn to navigate those dimensions, which the Tibetans call *bardo*, the "between," including the bardo of this world. Rumi, the great Sufi poet, describes "Body Intelligence" (Barks 1995, p. 151) in navigational terms:

You and your intelligence
Are like the beauty and precision
of an astrolabe.

Together, you calculate how near
Existence is to the sun!

Active Imagination

The genius of Avital's method is that it enables adults to recapture the faculty of active imagination that was so agile in childhood, and then use this power to slay old dragons of self-limitation and fear. Why are thresholds often so difficult to cross? Because imagined monsters lurk there, like trolls under a bridge, ready to turn the threshold into an obstacle. The workshop provides a rich environment in which to exercise the muscle of imagination and then walk upright again by means of it.

The root of *imagination* is *image* and we are inclined to think of images as visually static, like snapshots or icons. Guided visualization as accomplished in the mask session is a fully coordinated kinesthetic experience. Participants do not lie passively on the floor, they move as *act*-ors about the room. The session has the esthetic feel of Japanese Noh Theater. Imagination becomes an animating principle, not just a manipulation of mental objects. The distance between thought and action is compressed. Psychic space and physical space merge and one learns to navigate the terrain.

In *The Art of Memory*, Francis Yates describes the "inner gymnastics" of ancient bards and rhetors whose prodigious memories could retain thousands of lines of a poem or speech by assigning "places" to the lines in a carefully constructed "palace of memory." To retrieve the lines, the mental gymnast would return on an imaginative "tour" to the places where the lines were stored. (Yates 1974, p. 16) With the exception of a few contemporary memory experts, we have lost this capability.

We have also lost the ability, still possessed by some Micronesian sailors, to navigate long distances at sea without benefit of charts and instruments even when no landmarks are in view. Anthropologist Edwin Hutchins, in *Cognition in the Wild*, describes how such feats are accomplished. Micronesian navigators, instead of thinking of themselves as passing by objects on their way to a destination, conceive geography as streaming past the canoe. They have the astonishing ability to navigate by calculating great distances traveled past unseen reference points:

> Off to the side of the course being steered is the reference island…. Since the navigator has not actually *seen* the reference island at any point during the voyage, his ability to indicate where it lies represents an inference that could not be made in the Western system without recourse to tools. (Hutchins 1995, p. 72)

Hutchins explains that because Micronesian culture is non-literate, seafarers must memorize a large body of navigational information using "elaborate mnemonic devices." Even more interestingly, the Micronesian memory system makes "frequent reference to islands that do not exist." (Hutchins 1995, p. 73) The Micronesian navigates by an internal map. In essence, he is his own lodestar.

> In this system there are no universal units of direction, position, distance, or rate, no analog-to-digital conversions, and no digital computations. Instead, there are many special purpose units and an elegant way of "seeing" the world in which internal structure is superimposed on external structure to compose a computational image device. By constructing this image, the Micronesian navigator performs navigational computations in his "mind's eye." (Hutchins 1995, p. 93)

Although we live in a world of digital devices and digital computations, we easily lose our way. Like the Micronesian navigator seafaring with an inner astrolabe, we must learn again to use body intelligence to calculate "how near existence is to the sun."

Deep Orientation

The faculty of kinesthetic navigation or "deep orientation," as it plays a role in active imagination, goes far beyond the "inner gymnastics" Yates describes or Dennison's "Brain Gym" exercises. The feats of the Micronesian sailor do suggest, however, that we have far greater navigational skills than we might suspect.

One thing is clear: full-blown powers of active imagination manifested early in the drama of *homo sapiens*. In *Satyric and Heroic Mimes,* Kathryn Wylie compares how contemporary mimes resemble primordial shamans: both shaman and mime undergo rigorous corporeal training to develop a "repertoire of magical gestures"; both are known for trickster behavior; both use masks and pantomime to take on alternative identities and conjure objects and worlds out of thin air. (Wylie , 1994, p. 103)

Because mimicry is a natural human propensity—in fact many species practice mimesis as a survival strategy—it is impossible to say when the first "professional" performing mime appeared, but it is clear that shamans were among the earliest practitioners of the art:

> The shaman is a solo performer who undertakes the paradigmatic voyage of the mythical hero for the purpose of divination, exorcism, and curing. The events of the shaman's sacred voyage are frequently narrated gesturally in which corporeal images serve as metaphorical equivalents to the spoken or sung narration. Like modern day pantomimes who employ illusion, the shaman must make the invisible presences palpable for the audience by sleight-of-hand and manipulation of the laws of time and space. (Wylie , 1994, p. 7)

In contrast to passive notions of fantasy or daydreaming, this ability to conjure worlds in imagination, actively navigate those dimensions, and carry the knowledge across the threshold into the sun-lit world, is a powerful force—as demonstrated in Avital's mask session. Perhaps we fear that power. Perhaps that is why we resent the mime's frequent reminders that we live in an invisible three-dimensional box of our own making—and that we can step out of this self-created obstacle. But perhaps that is the ultimate object.

A version of this **"Afterword" "The Ultimate Object: Overcoming Self-Created Obstacles through Mime" has been published in the Journal of** *Bodywork & Movement Therapies***, Volume. 5, Number. 2. April, 2001, pp. 99-109. Published by Harcourt International.**

Jane Evenson has degrees in philosophy and literature. She works as a business consultant to support her explorations of kinesthetic intelligence and has known Samuel Avital and admired his work for close to nine years.

Jane Evenson may be contacted at jevenson@rmi.net.

References

Avital, Samuel 1985 Mime and Beyond: The Silent Outcry. Hohm Press, Prescott Valley, AZ

Barks, Coleman trans 1995 The Essential Rumi. HarperSanFrancisco, San Francisco

Cleary, Thomas and J. C. trans 1977 Blue Cliff Record, Vol. 3 Shambhala Publications, Boulder, CO

Gardner, Howard 1985 Frames of Mind. Basic Books, New York

Gleick, James 1993 Genius. Vintage Books, New York

Hannaford, Carla 1995 Smart Moves: Why Learning is Not All in Your Head. Great Ocean Publishers, Arlington, VA

Hiss, Tony 1990 The Experience of Place. Vintage Books, New York

Hutchins, Edwin 1995 Cognition in the Wild. The MIT Press, Cambridge, MA

Kaplan, Aryeh 1982 Meditation and Kabbalah. Samuel Weiser, York Beach, ME

Kurtzman, Joel 1999 An Interview with Howard Gardner. Strategy& Business 14: 90-99

Wilson, Frank R 1998 The Hand. Vintage Books, New York

Wylie, Kathryn 1994 Satyric and Heroic Mimes. McFarland & Company, Jefferson, NC

Yates, Francis 1974 The Art of Memory. The University of Chicago Press, Chicago

A P P E N D I X

The 8 Basic Principles of Conscious Integrated Being (CIB)

Here are eight practical insights to add to your practice. Keep them in your mind and heart with the focused daily exercise you are working at the time. Reflect and apply these principles and you'll witness the result of your dedication.

1. SMILE

Always smile. Smiling reverberates ALL the systems in your being and relaxes the whole body. The smile is not only in the face, but a natural reflection of happiness.

2. BREATHE

In every situation, observe the way you breathe. Be conscious of your breathing. Whenever you feel tension in any area of your body during any activity, remember to breathe. Breathing oxygenates the whole organism.

3. RELAXATION

Observe tensions in your jaw, neck, shoulders and pelvis. As soon as you become aware of tension in a specific area, remember to breathe and release. The more you practice this relatively simple technique, the better your body will learn by doing.

4. POSTURE

When walking, sitting or while doing any other activity, imagine seeing yourself in a mirror. LOOK at your posture. **KEEP THE SPINE STRAIGHT**. Ease the pressure from your abdominal area. Posture is the reflection of that which you are. Emotions condition our posture. Changing posture can change your emotions.

5. FOCUS

Focus your attention by listening to your breathing openly. Respond rather than react. Discover through focusing on an opportunity to learn something new about your self and how you function. Practicing this will make you discover the precious intimacy of this very moment of relating to your self and others.

6. MENTAL CONTROL

Observing reality **AS IT IS**, become aware of your thoughts as an observer, and the one who is being observed. Develop your mentality in a healthy, balanced way using your faculties of thinking creatively with no limitation. **SEEING THINGS AS THEY ARE** will become natural.

7. NOWNESS

Stay here now. Keep a constant attentiveness to this precious moment of being present. Feel and seize the full life power of this moment. Feel how the life force breathes and activates your being by always making you feel fully conscious of every moment. This is the only moment where you become aware of change, realizing who you are, keeping your visions and goals in mind and how to realize them. This ability of

NOWNESS assists you to integrate past with future into a potent and constant presence.

8. SILENCE

Being silent inside generates an immense force of energy. It is not only wise, but also a practical necessity to use silence in a world full of noise. This is a state of being I call, Le Centre du Silence. Speak less and do more. Speak ONLY when it is necessary. And even then, speak only that which is honest. Do not feel any pressure to talk. Small talk is a sign of emptiness. Silence enables you to increase the ability to listen and respond with only the amount of words necessary for expressing your self. When you practice this value of using silence, you will realize the power of being happy and productive - a sense of Super Happiness.

"Si ce que tu vas dire n'est pas plus beau que le silence ne le dis pas"
"If what you are going to say is not more beautiful than silence do not say it."
Anonymous

"We shall not cease from exploration and the end of all exploring will be
to arrive where we started and to know the place for the first time..."
T. S. Eliot

"Our culture is saturated with philosophical "Truths" that are commonly accepted and acted upon, and are rarely challenged. I think of these truisms as TRAPS. As long as they go unchallenged, they can keep you enslaved."
Harry Browne, How I Found Freedom In An Unfree World

"Great spirits have always encountered violent opposition from mediocre minds." **Albert Einstein**

"Be kind, for every one you meet is fighting a great battle"
Philo.

"What I desire I must sense, what I sense I create."
Michaelangelo

Body*Speak*™ WORKSHOP SERIES

This workshop series is designed and taught by Samuel Avital to introduce a way of observing and creatively practicing a totally integrated way of being, with a fresh view that will allow you to cause a positive change in your life. These descriptions are just a hint of the work you will be introduced to during your participation.

1. Live Long...Live Well: *The Art of Life Expansion*

The goal is not just to extend life but to expand it. Learn to feel and act younger and more vibrant. Expand your range of motion and activity. Enhance the quality of your life. Here are just a few of the proven body-mind techniques to be introduced and explored in depth during this intensive weekend:

THE LONGEVITY CYCLES
An innovative and highly effective series of rejuvenative exercises which integrate physical, mental, and emotional factors of being.

1. **The Flexibility Cycle**	is designed to gently limber and focus all parts of the body and
2. **The Regenerative Cycle**	integrates physical, mental and emotional attention to lubricate and regenerate the entire organism and
3. **The Integrative Cycle**	is a profound sequence to balance and focus your life force and theatrical skills.
4. **The Self-Evolutionary Cycle (4)**	is a practical series of ten (10) exercises to better your life, develop your balanced elf-guidance, and quicken your personal evolution.
The Moving Box Meditations	unique, artistic approach to meditation that enhances personal space awareness and which demonstrates that you don't have to sit still to calm the mind, reduce stress, and improve your ability to focus and concentrate.
Stop and Consider	attention-enhancing technique to sharpen the senses and extend the present.
Life-long Laughter	exercises exploring the role of humor and pleasure in life extension.

2. The Journey from Thought to Action: *Making the Invisible...Visible*

Jump into yourself. Un-block. Translate thoughts into words, bright ideas into action. Transform the ordinary into the extraordinary. Make the abstract, concrete. Improvise. Be spontaneous. Condense the time/space between thinking and doing. Tap your creative resources in a magical, entertaining, Body*Speak*™ learning event.

Here are some of the tools you'll wield:

Presentation without Words	**Act/React**
Shape-Shifter Improvisation	**Moving Box Meditation**
Stop-and-Consider	**Play it Again, Sam**
Apple Juggle	**Environmental Tableaux**
Moving Dragon	**Fish Story**

3. Personal Domain: *Being Present, Feeling Real, Making a Difference*

Domain: the state of being completely present, self-possessed, competent, able to effect action and influence outcomes. A true state of being as distinct from feelings of empowerment, which may be fleeting — especially if the power is actually bestowed by someone else. In this intensive weekend exploration of personal power, influence, and effectiveness, you will learn inventive body-mind methods for becoming the producer, director, and lead actor in your life. Write your own script ... starting NOW. Some topics we'll explore:

Presence	On developing a more compelling presence and expanding your "sphere of influence."
Personal Space	On gaining more command over your "local horizon" and personal security.
Authentic Expression	On feeling unique and real.
Attention	On getting and giving attention.

4. Touch Base: *The Art of Tenderness for Men and Women*

Women — and men — get weary. Try a little tenderness. Learn the art of Natural Gentle Touch™ (NGT) , sincere compliment, and pleasurable ritual. In a safe, inviting, and trusting environment, we'll explore:

The Snail Technique	The vehicle of Natural Gentle Touch: subtle, conscious, deliberate.
Compliments of the Chef	A great compliment is creative, precise, delicious, and well-done.
Windmill Meditation	Orientation via partner reflection.
Stop and Consider	Elasticizing the Present.
Foot/Earth Fascination	Bonding with gravity.
Subject/Object Relations	Entering the life of things.
Dialogue of the Hands	Rhythmic encounter of the hands.
The Sun/Moon Exercise	The interplay of opposites.
Tendriloquy™	The art of speaking, being and moving tenderly.

5. Walking the Line:
Exploring Personal Integrity and Authenticity through Movement

Daily living provides many challenges to our sense of personal integrity and authenticity. Through movement and group reflection, we will explore the essence of our individual being – both persona and mask:

The Zero	The center; starting point of all movement and decision; the integral plumb line.
The Edge	Crisis and transition; inclination of being.
Walking Against the Wind	The nature of struggle.
Bases	The foundation of physical and mental harmony.
Fixations	Deliberate, physical focus as a tool of precise and clear communication.
Parallels	For every action, there is an equal and opposite reaction.
Leaders and Followers	Proper functioning through balanced activity and passivity.
Animals and Elements	"Alert as a cat, fluid as water, still as a mountain."
Masks	A dramatic instrument to unleash the power of honesty and conscious choice.

6. The Walk of Power: *Mime for a New World*

Mimetic learning techniques are universally practiced in so-called "primitive" cultures but have been largely lost in Western Civilization. Usually by the time a child has reached adolescence, the inclination to joyful, spontaneous mimicry has been completely suppressed. "Don't be a copy cat," we say, "monkey see, monkey do." A tendency to conformism or group identification may be all that remains of the original delight in identifying with the natural world. A powerful source of creativity has dried up.

Actually, mimetic learning is not mere imitation. It is a **transformative art,** a method of capturing the essence of movement and a state of being by a powerful process of identification. This essence is fully embodied and represented through behavior. **Mime** is a vibrant means of extending the range of communicative behavior in both subtlety and   authentic power — of preserving our connection with nature and translating thought into action. The artist keeps this faculty alive. It has been said that "every creative genius is a specialized type of mime."

Body*Speak*™ is an ingenious method of reawakening the mimetic faculty — with profoundly beneficial results. Practice the art of state-shifting. Tap your creative resources in a magical **Body*Speak*™** learning event.

Here are some of the tools you'll learn to wield:

The Eye Compass	**Shape-Shifter Improvisation**
The Moving Box Meditation	**Environmental Tableaux**
The Paradoxical Windmill	**The Moving Dragon**
Handulations	**The Walk of Power**

7. Body*Speak*™ for Athletes: *Exploring "Deeper Will"*

This workshop is For private consultations and special group workshops. Please contact Le Centre Du Silence.

HERE'S WHAT PEOPLE ARE SAYING ABOUT
Samuel Avital and Body*Speak*™

Many of the endorsements and student testimonials included here are more like miniature essays, many gems, on the importance of mime and the art of movement in general. They are offered for the light they shed on the experiences of my students and in loving and mutual respect for the wisdom of colleagues and students alike and for all they have taught me over the years.—Samuel

▪▪

"I think that Samuel's work is important. He brings awareness to the soul of people and gives the young dedicated artists who work under his direction the need, dedication, and love for the world of silence and the beautiful art of movement. To my dear Samuel, words will always be poor beside our silence, but they will open doors to our silent spirit."

Marcel Marceau, BIP, 1976

"Mr. Avital is a remarkable man of astonishing depth and an artist of great magnitude and achievement, his profound knowledge of physical expression, teaching and performing is vast, rich and highly creative, his artistic fervor is contagious and his mastery is impeccable and practical... his method of teaching, is very well elaborated in his classic books. An inspired teacher, a magnetic, enthusiastic personality with excellent dedication and commitment."

Moni Yakim, Movement Theatre Director, Juilliard Drama Division, NYC. Author of "Creating a Character: A Physical Approach to Acting"

"Samuel Avital — whom I have known since his first years with my company in Paris — I suspected would become one of the great mimes. He has fulfilled that promise. He was among the first to reveal to me what creative interpretation could be, surpassing the creativity of the art of mime in order to become a human being who dares to be different.

"This great artist has discovered an extraordinary relationship between being an artist and becoming a true teacher of his own method. Our acquaintance has brought the greatest joy and surprise to my life and art."

Maximilien Decroux, Ecole Internationale de Mimodrame de Paris , Sept. 79

"Samuel Avital is an artist of conscious life, conscious theatre and cosmic laughter. When the madness of the world starts to get me down, I am lifted by the knowledge that men like Samuel exist. He remains unique, elusive, profound, demanding, dedicated, theatrical, passionate, and one of the most vibrant teachers I have encountered. Reveal your masks and his tools can peel them, reveal your heart and his tools are forever yours."

Mark Olsen, Summer student 1977. Assoc. Professor of Acting, Penn State, Univ. Park, PA. July 90

"Samuel Avital, founder and director of Le Centre Du Silence in Boulder, CO, has created a wondrous, spirited collection of essays, lectures, and exercises which explore not only the magical world of mime, but also the powerful integrating characteristics of art itself. While those interested in practicing mime will find this text to be an invaluable directive, Avital also presents a refreshing view of language, silence and movement **which appeal to the artist within us all...**

"...Both of Samuel's books have become classics and have contributed to the fruition of the American Theatre movement in the last few decades, such as the moon-walk of Michael Jackson, break dancing and the New Vaudevillians in the modern American theatre boom, and its holistic approach endears its ideas into the healing arts in America."

East West Journal, Review of *Mime & Beyond*, 1986

"Though Aristotle spoke of dancers who need neither poetry nor music, and such famous choreographers as Noverre, Folkine, Diaghilev, and Balanchine have used mimetic invention in ballet, the illusive art of mime did not come to America until Marceau brought it in 1955. It has grown in importance ever since.

"Samuel Avital, Director of Le Centre Du Silence Mime School, is one of the most interesting persons now teaching mime (and more). His *Mime Work Book* and *Mime & Beyond: The Silent Outcry*, originally written and used by Avital in the classroom, is now being read by teachers, actors, clowns, mimes, and dancers from coast to coast. **Universal in appeal,** it glows with Avital's personality."

American Dance Guild Book Club

"Have you ever seen the musical, 'My Fair Lady?' Remember how Colonel Pickering found it such a 'delightful challenge' to turn the 'poor, sniveling, crude, cockney flower girl,' Liza Doolittle into a 'real, live lady?' Her manners, speech, behavior, dress and total character were 'So wretched!' that the professor couldn't resist the challenge from his colleague to transform 'this thing! ' and pass her off as a Hungarian Duchess at a High Society Royal Ball. I loved watching the transformation of that poor, cockney flower girl into such a beautiful, graceful and elegant lady!

"This is the kind of transformation that I feel has been happening to me since I first started studying Body*Speak*™ with Samuel - Going from 'crude automechanical movements, ' to being 'at ease' with my body which has made me more confident in everything I do.

"What makes him so unique and special as a teacher? I like the fact that Samuel works from the premise that 'All human beings are intelligent and have the potential to be creative geniuses.' He believes in the individual. Working with him and studying Body*Speak*™ has helped me to realize and utilize my creative intelligence. He provokes one into breaking through limited mindsets, and helps to also activate full body intelligence. This frees one up to think and respond immediately in all kinds of situations.

"Another teacher quality that I find appealing in Samuel is, he gives personalized and individual attention. He addresses your needs and works with you towards realizing your goals. I have been gently nudged and sometimes forcibly pushed (playfully) to go beyond 'the edges' of my limited thinking and doing. Once 'pushed, ' new opportunities appear that I never thought of before.

"Body*Speak*™ is such a highly ordered and creative way to learn 'how to navigate in the world. ' No other form of education has ever matched the depth to which I have learned to discover new things about the body. Regular study of the Body*Speak*™ components, doing the exercise Cycles, and studying privately with Samuel, has helped me to 'properly ' direct, distribute and utilize creative energies.

"The work has not only helped me to develop my artistic qualities, but has also enhanced various skills in my professional career. I find that I handle any situation with calm and ease. I find that I can be totally involved in what I am doing at any given moment with passion, but a part of me can remain totally detached so that I can make rational and objective decisions.

"I have become a more independent and creative thinker, which helps me to make decisions with confidence. I find that I follow through with my actions, which is very important in my professional career.

"Communication skills have been enhanced and expanded in all areas. I am able to focus and concentrate to a higher degree on what I am doing which has lead me to be more energetic, creative and productive as a person.

"I have learned the art of responding rather than reacting. It is easier to stay balanced and centered in what I am doing. I continue to work with Samuel because I have found no other form of education to be as beneficial and easily applied in all situations. Life is more enjoyable and less hectic. I appreciate each new day as it comes.

"I would recommend that anyone who is wanting to change their life, sharpen their skills, would like some new tools for benefiting their personal and professional well-being, study Body*Speak*™ with Samuel. Body*Speak*™ is easily adaptable to all aspects of life and brings rich rewards!"

Alessandra, Caregiver in Nursing, Structural Integration Practitioner, Mime, Artist in Training and A Human "Becoming," Boulder, Colorado, Sunday March 28, 1999

"He was probably the single most influential teacher in my life. He teaches an excellent way to come into your own best fulfillment, with challenging ways of observing yourself and projecting yourself to others. In theatre, Samuel is an excellent place to start out and get a sense of what it really takes—from the inside out. For personal growth, **it is an experience you would value all your life.**"

Leslie Colket Blair, BMT 1973-1981. Editor/Actor/Writer/Singer

Samuel the simplest things become profound and important...**Every thought and action is scientifically pulled apart, and artistically integrated.** Samuel turns a fierce spotlight onto you. If you have the courage to be honest with yourself, you will begin to see new wonders."

Chris Hilder, Summer student 1990. Actor/Director, New Zealand

"He's intense, funny, severe, provocative, loving, compassionate and obnoxious. He's a teacher who gives his full range to his students. With Samuel, **I went from being a clumsy kid to an artist."**

Louis Greenstein, Actor/Playwright/Producer Boulder Mime Theatre 1978

"He is one of the most important people in my life. He helped crystallize becoming more aware of the responsibility of being an adult. He is relentless and doesn't accept compromises. He sees to the point quite lucidly. Any meeting with him sparks a response from him. If I were to recommend him to anyone I would say, 'do you want to change your life?'."

Sali Richardson, Photographer/Video Artist/Film Editor/Writer, 1978

"We move and don't know how we move. Samuel tries to slow movement down with different exercises. He was very helpful and took a special interest in me. He uses mime to work with people therapeutically. He was interested in me even though I was such a beginner"

Susan Rangitsch, Summer student 1989, Transpersonal Therapist

"He teaches things that you couldn't find anywhere else. You create stories through your body to show off a particular skill and go far beneath that. He has an impact on people through performance."

Rachel McCaleb, Full-time Mother. Boulder Mime Theatre 1976-1977

"I learned to trust my body to honestly express itself. As a result of the workspace, I have become comfortable with my body, to acknowledge past blocks, release them, and open to new horizons. I also realize that it is I, alone, who limit myself, and it's up to me to exercise my inner power of my own authority in personal encounters, especially when expressing my convictions."

Marie Fuchik , Maple Heights, OH

"I had come to a point in my life where I was totally confused, and needed both artistically and personally, a new, better way of looking at life. I learned many principles and movements, how to let my body's natural honesty influence my mind...the first steps to total integration. It will take time for me to duly realize the mastery of anatomical alchemy that is Mime. My appetite has been 'enflamed'."

John Biedenbach, Trenton, MI

"I came to Samuel's workspace because I was in a transition period in my life, and wanted to take a risk and do something different. I learned that I am always the cause of my pain, and that I am the only one who stand in my way. Samuel presents many universal truths in his teaching. He is very intense, but workable. I would like to study more with Samuel either in workshops or individually."

Ana Calantini, Mt. Shasta, CA

"I have learned and affirmed that there is nothing I need to hide from myself. In being honest with myself, my communication with others is enhanced. My true self knows my direction. No obstacles need to be created. The true path can be revealed at any moment when distractions do not keep me from it. In my truth is freedom."

Justine Cahn Fenu, Syracuse, NY

"Be prepared to surrender to yourself! Samuel strips us to the core to wake us up. He helps us to close the gap between thought and action, making us realize that we are more conscious and integrated beings.."

Shannon McCarthy, Montrose, CO

"Oh, Samuel, you are magic! I move totally differently. I am conscious about my behavior. The workshop has helped me stay more focused on what I want to do, how to relate to different people and to experience honesty in mind and body. *BodySpeak*™ techniques have helped me appreciate much more larger things, the bigger picture of what I want to do, to be and become"

Valentina Vargas, Actor, Hollywood, CA , Summer student, July 93

"I gained a perspective on the artistic beauty that is inside me, and want to bring this artistic and creative self into relationship with others, and the world...The approach to using "the body" as a metaphor for relating to the world is a very sound approach to living."

David George, Boulder, CO, Dec 93

"Body*Speak*™ Workshop is the powerful self-revolution that helps me to govern myself with my own authority. It will provide you with the most honest tools of communication to better relate to yourself and your environment."

Béatrice Du Jardin, Paris, France , Jan 93

"Working with Samuel is somewhat like being the overcurious sorcerer's apprentice. Enticed by the deceptive simplicity of the work, I dive in and suddenly find myself drowning in a flood, with brooms marching endlessly back and forth carrying even more buckets of water to douse me. In the nick of time, the flood subsides. The Mimagician returns, grabs me by a soggy collar and we turn back to page one in the Book of Silence... .My teacher is a big ring of invisible keys —they dangle in my hands as I stand before as many unmarked invisible doors. There is no superficiality here. To slide easily on the surface of mime-form would be a betrayal of this art."

Dorothy Ormes, Story teller, Chico, CA. Summer student 1978

"Samuel has created simple tools that absolutely awaken the spirit and ground the body. Each learner is initiated into the reality that coded in the physical body are key principles for living a creative and purposeful life. He is a grandfather in this field of using conscious movement for one's inner practice."

Melissa Michaels, Movement Educator, Boulder, CO , Feb 94

"Samuel begins at the point of creation and proceeds to manifest world upon world. Spirit, Mind and Body are his tools to mold form from space. My work with Samuel over the years has been a great inspiration in my life."

Pamela Rose-Kier, Midwife, actress, Boulder, CO Mar 94

"Cyclists move through a limited range of motion and there fore become physically unbalanced— even un- coordinated—over time. I found that by studying and participating in different types of movement disciplines during my career, I was able to develop coordination and flexibility, as well as to build strength. Additionally, it was refreshing to do something different. I found Samuel Avital's approach to movement to be intriguing, informative, and very useful. It's good work for the body...and the soul."

Connie Carpenter, Olympic Cyclist, Boulder CO , Mar 94

"I have been running long distance for about 3 years, running in general for 15 years. When I increased my mileage to runs averaging 25 to 30 miles in length, I encountered barriers which I experienced as pain or discomfort or fatigue. I have worked on my internal development enough to realize that these barriers had as much to do with emotional and mental attitudes as with the physical challenge itself.

"In working with Samuel, I have gained a deeper understanding and body knowledge of how thought, feeling, and body work as a unit. I feel lighter, less inhibited, more playful. My body is more supple and fluid. I have become more aware of how energy flows in my body. My movement has become more directed and organized, and I run with less effort. Best of all, *I* make the decision to be running this way now. Before I would have the experience randomly or accidentally. I feel more self-confident. I have developed a deeper will."

Melissa Huntress, Long distance runner, Boulder, CO, Feb 94

"Avital's work reaches beyond theater arts, to explore the reality of physical embodiment. Practitioners of the somatic arts will find much of great value in his teaching, for deepening and expanding both vision and practical effectiveness in their work. I have worked with Samuel's classes, and found that there are many parallels between the approach he teaches and that of Structural Integration."

Peter Melchior, Rolfer, Guild for Structural Integration, Inc. Boulder, CO, Mar 94

"I have found the work of Samuel Avital to be tremendously helpful in my activities, I must often convey complex scientific concepts to funding agencies and fellow researchers, and understand and using non-verbal communications is critical to transmitting such ideas.

"I have also found it enriches my practice of NLP (Neuro-Linguistic-Programing) psychotherapy and communication."

Robert B. Owen, B.S., PhD. (physics). M.A., PhD. (Anthropology) Certified NLP Master Practitioner. Mar 94

"Samuel Avital works and teaches his students with the same totally involved detachment with which Horowitz addresses the piano."

Pasty Swank, Dallas Magazine, Nov 1969

"I find Samuel Avital's work to be a delightful complement to the Feldenkrais Method. I highly recommend this class to my friends and students."

Jack Heggie, The Boulder Center for the Feldenkrais Method®, Author of *Running with the Whole Body* and *Skiing with the Whole Body,* Boulder, Colorado 1994.

"Until Samuel Avital's class (1971) I don't believe I had ever experienced by own ability to improvise. Once I did, I found a lifelong skill tapped, released, and utilized to this day... over 27 years later. As Samuel so eloquently says, "the Body Speaks" — a metaphor, once learned through the kind of training that M. Avital offers, that becomes an incredibly useful tool in one's personal as well as professional life.

"I credit Mr. Avital with helping me develop a keener sense of myself and, as important, a more watchful and intuitive sense of the people around me. I believe what he offers is extremely valuable, and appropriate, to people in leadership capacities."

Lois LaFond singer/songwriter, Boulder, CO

"In the summer of 1985, I was 16 years old and I attended a month-long workshop led by Samuel Avital. Fourteen years later, I still find that I refer back to what I learned and experienced with Samuel and it continues to inspire, interest, and assist me in many aspects of my professional and personal life.

"I feel Samuel's work contributed greatly to my sense of, and comfort in, my own body. As a dancer, singer and future medical practitioner, this is extremely essential. His workshop helped me in establishing a solid base from which I draw strength and confidence when I am performing to an audience, teaching a class and interacting with people on a one-to-one basis.

"I also am greatly appreciative of how Samuel shares his wisdom with his students. I recall vividly how I felt empowered during and after the workshop. I returned home feeling a strong sense of purpose and direction in my life. What I learned from Samuel has endured over time. When I review over the work we did during that month, I am again imbued with a sense of balance, depth and gratitude.

"I consider studying with Samuel Avital to be a great opportunity for people of all ages and disciplines. I would highly recommend his classes to students of all ages and professions.

Deborah Savran, Singer, Dancer and Dance Teacher,and Natural Medicine Student, April 7, 1999

"It is difficult to count the many benefits I received under your tutelage. Today, I am a successful businessman, President of my own executive search firm. We recruit and place executives into important positions with major corporations around the country.
The most important learning you provided was related to "body language," and I have used this intuitive knowledge throughout my career. You taught very clearly: "The body does not lie!" I have found this to be true. When I interview an executive or manager, I can tell instantly whether they are telling me the truth, whether they have the stamina and integrity required for the job.

"I cannot thank you enough for your influence on me when I was but a wide-eyed student. My creative drive, my leadership skills, my sensitivity to others, and my love of the arts were also greatly enhanced during my two years of study with you.

"I hope that hundreds more students have the chance to study with you, to receive the many gifts you have to bear. You have my gratitude and my best wishes for your continued success and happiness."

Lion Goodman, Mill Valley, CA

"I have been impressed with your devotion to the art of mime and especially to the art of Living. You have combined the vigorous study of mime with the importance of living ethically.

"Many of the students who have studied with you have told me how wonderful working with has been.'

Tony Montanaro, Montanaro/Hurll Theatre of Mime and Dance, Paris, Maine, USA, March 15, 1999

"It is with pleasure that I extend this support letter for Samuel Avital. His life work has always been, and remains to this day, completely dedicated to helping the individual emerge strong, focused, and dynamically engaged in life. He demands clarity of thought and action from each student and through humor, example, and precise, physically engaging exercises, guides them to a state of personal growth and self-authority. They literally begin to assume the authorship of their own lives.

"There are few teachers and guides who have the integrity and capacity to promote healthy leadership. Most use their enthusiasm to charm and induce the student into assuming a predigested program of study that does little more than promote a temporary false confidence. Samuel's teaching goes directly to the heart of each person, challenging them to formulate their vision with unflinching honesty, chart their action with verve, take responsibility for their choices with relish, and then to free their imaginative powers from the conditioned self-imposed restrictions.

"In my own life, Samuel's teachings have helped me to assume responsibilities of greater and greater demand - all with a sense of humor and grace. I have become a respected teacher and leader in my own field, passing on many of the core ingredients I first absorbed from Samuel over twenty years ago. His words, his life, his teaching, his writings, have all contributed to the foundation upon which I have built my life work.

"I am not alone in this estimation of Samuel's contributions. His work has a long legacy of successful students who are today working in all facets of our society and at all levels, fearlessly confronting the challenges of life. They all received from him what he most freely gives: the space, time, and tools to break out of their shell and live a bold, self-directed life.

"I commend anyone who has the foresight to link his or her work with Samuel's. His methods and delicious sense of vivacity can breathe new life into any project, program, or work, extending the potential of all involved and rooting the growth in a sane, integrated, process. Please give Samuel Avital your utmost consideration and be assured that his involvement will meet and far exceed your expectations.

Mark Olsen, Associate Professor - Penn State School of Theatre, Penn State Univ. University Park, PA, 1999

"It is my pleasure to recommend Samuel Avital, Founder and Director of Le Centre du Silence to any business, educational, or technical organization which needs to develop an effective organization using innovative transformational leadership technologies, dynamic learning skills, and individual and organizational empowerment strategies.

"Over the years, I have experienced Mr. Avital's personal and professional commitment to excellence. He has provided insightful and useful assistance, consulting, and coaching to myself in the areas of leadership development, strengthening of will, regeneration of a sense of purpose, direction in my life, and clarification of goals and strategic actions.

"He has greatly benefited my personal and professional well being. Specifically, I have noted his ability to target and get to the core truth of an issue I may have been challenged by. In doing so, it has provided me with a focused and direct direction in dealing with these issues. I have also been impressed with his passion and compassion in my relationship with him.

"I would have to say, from my experience, that Mr. Avital is a unique person of immeasurable substance and wisdom who has and will continue to capture the essence of true individual and organizational success."

Gary Goldman, President International Quality Leadership Institute, Chicago, IL

"Taught and developed by Samuel Avital, director of Le Centre du Silence, Body*Speak*™ encourages and challenges growth in every student who learns its principles. This growth in creativity and personal understanding extends beyond art and deep into one's being. Learning mime from Samuel Avital is learning about life. A student of the Avital's method studies principles. These principles, learned within the framework of mime, create powerful analogies to life itself. These analogies foster insight about who we are and how we live. The same, Body*Speak*™ principles used to create elegance in our bodies help create beauty within our lives.

"Through Avital's method, mime becomes a tool to help build and maintain a fuller life.

"Samuel's principles foster self-reliance within our busy sometimes-jumbled world. As a mime's feet stand firmly on the stage ready to move and create, a Le Centre du Silence student learns to stand firmly in the world ready to create and live fully. Samuel's principles empower each individual to embrace life. Students are encouraged to push to the edge of life—without falling. Learning to trust oneself and listen to one's own voice are empowering forces needed within this world.

"As a mime, Samuel Avital's classroom opened my eyes to new, beautiful aspects of the silent art. As an individual, Samuel's principles enriched my life. The principles that improved my art extended beyond the studio and stage and into life itself. The art I love helped me carve a more holistic place in this world. Samuel helps people find their dance on the world's stage.

"Learning mime with Samuel Avital calls for one to reflect, to question, to ponder, and to risk. The reflection fosters insight; the questions encourage understanding, the pondering leads to enlightenment, and the risks lead to immeasurable rewards. It is impossible to learn only mime and movement at Le Centre du Silence. At this school of mime, enriched, more holistic life is always the topic and always the goal."

Tim Chartier, Mime, and puppeteer, Boulder, Colorado

"Like the art of its teacher, Avital's method is beyond words. Describing Samuel's classroom calls for imagery and shape. In an effort to describe the teaching of Samuel Avital, I turn to the Body*Speak*™ logo and its use of contrasts.

"For a moment, look at the picture. Notice the curves, the lines, the contrasts, the separateness, and the wholeness. The picture calls the viewer to look at the differences and yet, the image is a collected whole.

"Now that you have looked at the image, let me describe Samuel's workshop within this imagery.

"Samuel teaches through contrasts—from understanding to misunderstanding, from risk to safety, from comfort to struggle, from failure to success. The contrasts are often stark. Still, there is a cycle to the contrasts; there is a flow and a rhythm. We undulate from safety to risk to safety again. We float from struggle to comfort to struggle. The pattern is intentional and still spontaneous and personal. Like drops of water in a river, we flow on our own paths. Some drops find quick currents and others discover contemplative, placid pools. At the same time, we form a community, a unison, and a connectedness. We flow together toward something unseen. Yet all along, the river seems to know the direction.

"Samuel searches the individual. Like the image, his eyes are open. He looks at you, around you, and into you. He offers the same for his students. He shares himself—his humor, his depth, his opinions, and his learnings. Samuel calls for honesty and openness. He strives to find the core—of the learning, of the individual, and of the community. To succeed, we all must be attentive, awake, ready, and searching. For in any moment, life can unfold quickly and subtly. We must be ready and alert to see the truths and nuances.

"Samuel Avital offers a classic image of teaching where the learner is free to learn, free to discover, and free to explore. He searches for the simplest avenue to the destination. The path is so direct that he sometimes doesn't even offer us a map. He extends his gentle hands and simply calls us to come, to follow, to play, to dance, as well as to silence.

"Samuel's teaching calls you whoever you are, whatever your interests, and whatever your path. He offers an environment to discover yourself in a fuller, creative way. He asks that you come with your light and darkness, with your edges and curves. He calls you to come as you. If you want to learn, come ready to teach. If you come to receive, be ready to give. If you come to connect with others, be ready to connect with yourself. Yet, no matter your goals, your wishes, your dreams, I believe Samuel offers avenues for you to reach for your stars in new ways. Why do I say this? Samuel Avital searches for an environment in which each of us can find ourselves, knowing that he, himself, will also grow — and through the process we learn together in community."

Tim Chartier , Mime, and puppeteer, Boulder, Colorado
"As I reflect on Samuel Avital and his teaching, many things come to mind...
As a middle school reading and drama teacher, I can recognize many ways in which Samuel Avital's workshop has impacted me. I am present within my task, awake and ready to write/plan lessons that will teach my students some of the very concepts that I just have learned. I am excited to help them recognize the amazingly complex, yet simple, connection between the body and the mind.

"The dichotomous learning that frequently goes on in classrooms has been a frustration for me for quite some time, and I have worked to expand my repertoire of kinesthetic learning activities. Your workshop has contributed greatly to this. I have already incorporated Leader/Follower and The Great Puzzle into my plans and am working at using portions of the cycles for warm-up and focusing activities.

"Many people will think it natural that I incorporate mime exercises into drama, but may be surprised that I truly believe that my reading students will benefit as much or more. I will utilize Leader/Follower as a model for the use of reading strategies. Just as people don't often think of leading their walk with the elbow or the chin, many of my students don't think of using the various reading strategies, such as highlighting or graphic organizers, to make meaning from their reading. It all depends on the purpose and what one is trying to get out of the text — be it the body or the written word. I find the beauty of mime reveals many things that can be taught within the world of words.

"From my perspective as a student in this workshop, I have learned much about the beauty behind the integrated art of mime. The essence of mime is something I understand to a better degree than before the workshop. I have often been able to sense an artist at work within technique, but knew that technique only was not the answer to the deep messages that came forth from the art. Technique is essential; however, it cannot communicate without the artist being wholly present and within the moment. I now find myself more focused and expressive within simple movement. I believe I am learning about myself as well as mime.

"This workshop was an experience of inquiry into the body and what it means to live in full recognition of the body, not simply in spite of it. I feel more connected to myself and am amazed at how giving attention to my entire body can help it health-wise."

Tanya Chartier, Reading/Theatre Teacher, Mime, Clown, Boulder, CO

"I attended the 26th International Summer Mime Workshop July 1997 run by Samuel Avital. What attracted me to attend was that the workshop was not merely teaching a mime technique, but also a new and fresh way of looking at the self and life. I had come from a spiritual background where I had learned to develop increased self confidence, an inner stability, an overall positive outlook and a mental calm in my approach to life and its many situations, enabling me to feel that anything was possible, and that it all depended on me.

"When I attended Samuel Avital's workshop I was delighted to find that through his method of teaching mime and asking the student to reflect on the process that was taking place inside the self and looking at how one would use that experience in practical situations, in connection with the physical technique being taught, gave me a very similar experience, and it was so refreshing to be coming to very similar conclusions and realizations, and new ones, from a completely different approach.

161

"Samuel has a very alive approach to life and, along with the technique he has developed, he brings a lot of life and laughter to the sessions, allowing a great openness among the participants which creates an opportunity for deep personal growth to take place within the short period of the workshop. This is always a necessity when it comes to developing leadership qualities and inner strength, as you are given a chance to look deeply at the self.

"I found that on returning I was re-energized mentally and physically, with a renewed sense of purpose and direction in my life, and with methods at hand to sustain the process."

Pamela Baillie, Secretary with the World Health Organization, Geneva, Switzerland 1999

"With his method of Body*Speak*™, Samuel Avital offers a concrete physical embodiment of his philosophical teachings.

"Through physical application during Samuel's workshop, I learned of the innate intelligence of both body and universe, and thus found the confidence to take necessary risks, and to travel beyond the 'edge. ' By studying 'motion/stillness' I discovered that purposeful action can take hold in an instant, allowing me to avoid the paralysis of procrastination. Problems that seemed unsolvable offered their own solutions once I experienced my body's reaction to 'fixation.' Through Samuel's many applications I learned to take responsibility for my own creativity ability, to be a script maker—not a script follower. Samuel's movement 'cycles' taught me the importance of discipline and conscious awareness.

"Through Samuel's teachings, I have become aware of what my body says to others, and what my body says to me. My mind watches my body; my body reflects my mind. Thus (through the work Samuel offers) I am offered a mirror with which I can see myself."

Gregg Tobo, Research Analyst, Storage Tek, Boulder, CO, April 1, 1999

"I had the opportunity of working with Samuel Avital when I was a young adult in 1970-71 in Boulder, Colorado, at a very important juncture in my life. I had left college after three years in the tumultuous 1960s and was seeking experiences that would better direct me toward both career decisions and personal satisfaction. I was extremely fortunate to have discovered Samuel and Le Centre Du Silence Mime School.

"It was while working with Samuel that I recognized not only my passion for performance but for collective, ensemble work — work that I continue to do to this day as a practitioner of the techniques of theatre director and social activist Augusto Boal (Theatre of the Oppressed), and as a professor at California Institute of the Arts. Samuel taught me how to focus my attention, how to be sensitive to the movement and desires of others around me, how to dialogue with space, and perhaps most importantly, how to be manifest my own movements and desires through space, through life. Samuel helped launch my confidence in a way that no one had up until that point. I remain forever grateful for his dedication, strength, craft, generosity, and leadership. I am particularly grateful for his rare ability as a teacher to inspire the development of all of these qualities in others.

"I am currently a writer with several articles published and my second book on its way. Besides my work as a full time teacher, I am Assistant Dean in the School of Critical Studies at CalArts and active in several organizations dedicated to the integration of art and social change. I think of Samuel Avital as my first teacher, though so many teachers had come before him. I truly believe my time studying with him was a very special time studying my own potential, through the guidance of a very potent teacher indeed."

Mady Schutzman, Assistant Dean and Professor School of Critical Studies - California Institute of the Arts - March 28, 1999

"I'm writing to recommend the remarkable talents of Samuel Avital. Over the years, I have taken several of his wonderful courses and workshops. During that period, was transitioning from my career as a lawyer to becoming a Certified *Feldenkrais*® Practitioner? Samuel's work combines some of the best qualities of both of my professions.

"The people in Samuel's groups have a broad range of cognitive skills, intelligence and education. Most also have their creative side. Samuel's gift is his ability to teach us to combine these qualities through the use of mime. He brings out his students their dynamic expressive side by the use of his wonderful mind-body work. He is a master.

"For me, the most important aspect I took away was the process for expressing my creative side through a body dynamic. That process is with me still, as I now teach others to move dynamically and expressively through my own method in my own practice. I'll never forget the many things I learned through working with Samuel. He is a person of high caliber with a rare and special skill."

Jan K. Bernstein, Certified *Feldenkrais*® Practitioner, Denver, CO

Samuel Avital

BIOGRAPHY OF SAMUEL AVITAL

The early years of Samuel Avital's life were set in a small village Sefrou, near Fez, in the Atlas Mountains of Morocco. Educated in the home of a simple but unique family, which traces its lineage back many years, carrying from father to son, in the Sephardic tradition the ancient and beautiful practical wisdom of the Hebrew Kabbalah.

At the age of 14, Samuel traveled to Israel where he spent a ten years, living in a kibbutz and other schools. He studied physics, agronomy, theology, arts and theatre.

His innate interest in the arts eventually drew him to Paris where he studied dance and theatre at the Sorbonne. Here he discovered the world of mime in the teachings of the master, Etienne Decroux.

Having met his art form, Avital threw himself into what he found to be the very essence of human expression. Decroux, Barrault, and Marceau were all to have a profound influence on the formation of his own artistic expression. He soon began touring with Maximilien Decroux and performing his own solo performance.

In 1964, Samuel joined his friend Moni Yakim in New York, performing with Yakim in his Pantomime Theatre of New York and also in off off-Broadway theatres, as well as teaching mime in the New York City schools. Later, he toured in North and South America and Canada, and in 1969 he was invited to teach at SMU in Dallas.

In 1971 he established **Le Centre du Silence Mime School** in Boulder, Colorado. The following year he created the **Boulder Mime Theatre** with his most dedicated students. The **BMT** performed during the next 12 years in local, state and national engagements.

In 1975 Avital initiated the International Summer Mime Workspace, an annual intensive course attracting students worldwide. The same year he published his *MIME WORKBOOK* followed by a second edition in 1977, a third printing in 1982, and *MIMENSPIEL,* a German edition out of Frankfurt. Hohm Press, Prescott, Arizona, published his second book, *MIME & BEYOND: The Silent Outcry* in 1985. *The Conception Mandala* by Samuel Avital and Mark Olsen was published by Inner Traditions, Rochester, VT. His video, *The Silent Outcry: The Life and Times of Samuel Avital* was produced in 1992. In 1985 he was nominated for the Colorado Governor's Award for Excellence in the Arts.

Over the years he developed his unique method of teaching, and created Body*Speak*™. He has also contributed numerous articles, interviews and essays in several languages to diverse publications throughout the U.S. and abroad. Currently Avital lives in Boulder, Colorado where he continues his artistic activities, and offers his seminars and workshops in the US and Europe.

For more information and program training, write, call, email or visit the Le Centre du Silence Web site.

Le Centre du Silence Mime School, Samuel Avital. Director.
P.O. Box 1015 (TBSM) Boulder, Colorado, 80306-1015 – (303) 662-9271
Email: savital@concentric.net
Website: http://www.indranet.com/lcds.html

About the Author

Samuel Avital was born in the town of Sefrou near the Atlas mountains in Morocco. In 1958, he moved to Paris to study with the masters of mime – Etienne Decroux, and Marcel Marceau. In 1971, he **founded Le Centre du Silence Mime School** in Boulder, Colorado. In addition to performing internationally, he also holds workshops on Mime and kinesthetic expression *BodySpeak*™, teaches privately, and hosts a bi-weekly forum of creative expression called **Café-Salon Philosophique**. In addition to numerous articles, Avital has published three book – "**Mime Workbook**" (1975) (a German edition, "**Mimenspiel**" was published in 1985), "**Mime and Beyond: the Silent Outcry**" (1985), and "**The Conception Mandala**: Creative Techniques for Inviting a Child into Your Life" (1992), co-authored with Mark Olsen. His life and work are also the subject of a video, "**The Silent Outcry: the Life and Times of Samuel Avital.**"

CPSIA information can be obtained at www.ICGtesting.com
Printed in the USA
BVOW06s1027110214

344598BV00006B/511/A